RENALDIET COOKBOOK FOR SENIORS

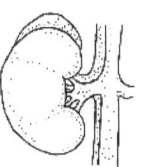

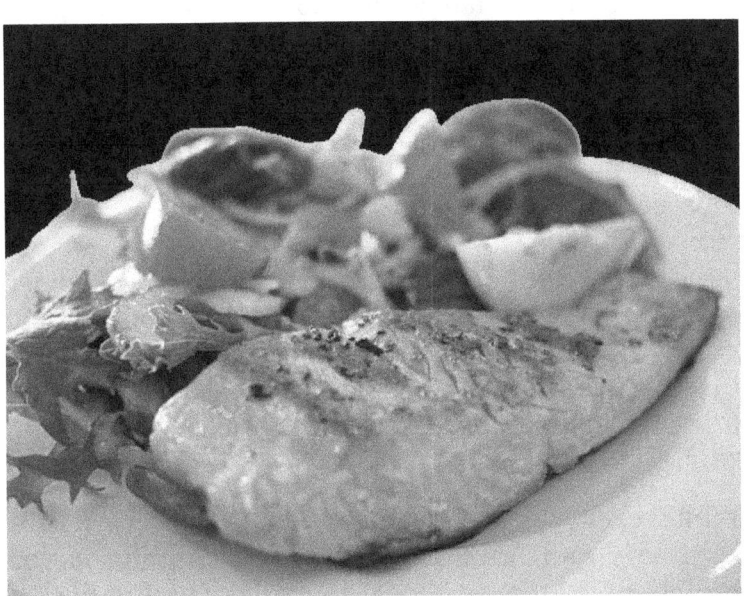

The complete easy, nutritious, tasty recipes for managing kidney disease, a healthy and vibrant you in your golden years.

BRENDA.M. SMITH

Copyright © 2024 BY BRENDA.M. SMITH

This cookbook is intended to give information and recipes for those following a renal diet. The author and publisher are not engaged in providing medical advice or services. The information in this cookbook should not be used as a substitute for professional medical care or guidance. Consult a certified healthcare practitioner for tailored advice based on your health situation.

While every effort has been made to ensure the accuracy and completeness of the information presented in this cookbook, the author and publisher assume no responsibility for errors or omissions, misuse, or damages resulting from the use of the information contained herein.

TABLE OF CONTENT

INTRODUCTION

A Cookbook for Seniors on the Renal Diet"! This cookbook is more than just a collection of recipes; it's a culinary companion designed specifically for older adults navigating the challenges of kidney-related health issues. Whether you're managing chronic kidney disease (CKD), kidney stones, or kidney failure, this cookbook supports you on your journey to better kidney health.

Our bodies change as we age, and our nutritional needs evolve. For seniors facing kidney issues, maintaining a balanced diet becomes paramount in managing their condition and enhancing their quality of life. That's where the renal diet comes in—a specialized eating plan designed to alleviate the strain on the kidneys by regulating the intake of certain nutrients.

But following a renal diet doesn't mean sacrificing flavor or satisfaction. It's quite the opposite. With this cookbook, you'll discover a world of delicious, kidney-friendly recipes that prove you don't have to compromise on taste to support your kidney health. From hearty soups and stews to vibrant salads and satisfying mains, each recipe is thoughtfully crafted to be nutritious and delicious.

This cookbook is more than just a collection of recipes; it's a comprehensive guide to easily navigating the renal diet. Inside, you'll find practical tips for meal planning, ingredient substitutions, and dining out, ensuring that you can enjoy flavorful, satisfying meals wherever you go. Plus, you'll learn about the principles of the renal diet and how to tailor your eating habits to support your kidney health.

Whether you're cooking for yourself or loved ones, this cookbook is your go-to resource for nourishing, kidney-friendly meals that will delight your taste buds. So grab your apron and prepare to embark on a culinary journey that nourishes both body and soul. Here's to delicious food, vibrant health, and happy cooking!

Understanding the Renal Diet: A Guide for Seniors

The renal diet is a customized eating regimen that promotes kidney health and helps those with kidney disease. This diet focuses on managing the consumption of key nutrients such as sodium, potassium, phosphorus, and protein to regulate the workload of the kidneys and maintain optimal function. The renal diet tries to relieve stress on the kidneys, control fluid balance, and minimize waste product buildup in the circulation by carefully monitoring these factors. This dietary strategy is critical in sustaining overall kidney function and increasing the quality of life for those who have renal problems.

"Understanding the Renal Diet: A Guide for Seniors" is not just another dietary resource; it's a lifeline for older adults facing the challenges of kidney-related health issues. Imagine having a comprehensive guide tailored specifically to your needs, offering clear, practical advice on how to manage your diet to support kidney health and overall well-being.

Our bodies undergo various changes as we age, and our nutritional requirements evolve. For seniors grappling with kidney conditions like chronic kidney disease (CKD) or kidney failure, the importance of a renal diet cannot be overstated. This specialized eating plan is not just about what to eat; it's about empowering seniors to take control of their health and improve their quality of life.

The beauty of "Understanding the Renal Diet: A Guide for Seniors" lies in its simplicity and accessibility. It breaks down complex dietary information into easy-to-understand principles, ensuring that seniors can grasp the concepts and implement them with confidence. From practical meal planning tips to delicious, kidney-friendly recipes, this guide provides everything seniors need to navigate the intricacies of the renal diet with ease. It is a guide that shows seniors that they can still enjoy flavorful, satisfying meals while adhering to the renal diet, ensuring that their culinary experiences remain a source of joy and pleasure.

Importance of Nutrition in Kidney Health

Managing Kidney Function: Certain nutrients can directly impact kidney function. For example, excessive intake of sodium, potassium, and phosphorus can strain the kidneys and exacerbate conditions like chronic kidney disease (CKD). By following a balanced diet tailored to their specific needs, individuals with kidney issues can help preserve their kidney function and slow the progression of kidney disease.

Preventing Complications: Poor nutrition can increase the risk of complications associated with kidney diseases, such as fluid retention, electrolyte imbalances, bone disorders, and cardiovascular problems. A well-planned diet can help prevent these complications by controlling nutrient intake and supporting overall health.

Managing Symptoms: Kidney disease and its treatments can cause various symptoms that affect appetite, digestion, and nutrient absorption. A dietitian can help individuals with kidney issues develop a meal plan that addresses these symptoms and ensures adequate nutrition to support overall well-being.

Controlling Blood Pressure: High blood pressure is a common complication of kidney disease and can further damage the kidneys. A diet low in sodium and rich in fruits, vegetables, and whole grains can help lower blood pressure and reduce the risk of cardiovascular complications.

Supporting Bone Health: Kidney disease can disrupt the body's ability to balance calcium and phosphorus levels, leading to weakened bones and an increased risk of fractures. Adequate calcium and vitamin D intake, along with phosphorus restriction as needed, can help maintain bone health in individuals with kidney issues.

Promoting Overall Health: Good nutrition is essential for overall health and well-being, especially for individuals with kidney disease. A balanced diet that provides essential nutrients, vitamins, and minerals supports the body's immune function, energy levels, and overall vitality.

How This Cookbook Can Help You

Provides Kidney-Friendly Recipes: A renal diet cookbook offers a wide variety of recipes that are specifically tailored to meet the dietary restrictions of individuals with kidney issues. These recipes are designed to be lower in sodium, potassium, phosphorus, and protein, making it easier to plan meals that support kidney health.

Offers Nutritional Information: Renal diet cookbooks often provide nutritional information for each recipe, including details on sodium, potassium, phosphorus, and protein content. This allows you to make informed decisions about which foods to include in your meal plan and how to balance your nutrient intake.

Saves Time and Effort: Planning meals can be challenging, especially following a specialized diet. A renal diet cookbook takes the guesswork out of meal planning by providing a collection of kidney-friendly recipes that you can easily reference whenever you need inspiration.

Promotes Variety: Following a renal diet doesn't mean you have to eat the same foods every day. A renal diet cookbook offers a wide range of recipes, from soups and salads to main dishes and desserts, allowing you to enjoy a diverse and flavorful diet while still adhering to your dietary restrictions.

Encourages Healthy Eating Habits: Renal diet cookbooks often emphasize whole, nutrient-rich foods like fruits, vegetables, whole grains, and lean proteins. By incorporating these foods into your diet, you can improve your overall nutrition and support your kidney health.

Empowers You to Take Control: Having access to a renal diet cookbook empowers you to take control of your diet and make choices that support your kidney health. With a variety of delicious recipes at your fingertips, you can feel confident knowing that you're taking proactive steps to manage your condition and improve your quality of life.

CHAPTER 1: RENAL DIET BASIC

What is chronic kidney disease {CKD}?

Chronic kidney disease (CKD) is a long-term condition where the kidneys gradually lose their function over time, typically progressing through stages of severity. To understand CKD, it's essential to grasp the role of the kidneys in the body.

Kidney Function:

The kidneys are vital organs responsible for filtering waste products, excess fluids, and toxins from the blood, which are then excreted as urine.

They help regulate electrolyte levels, such as sodium, potassium, and calcium, which are critical for maintaining fluid balance, nerve function, and muscle contraction.

The kidneys also produce hormones that regulate blood pressure, stimulate red blood cell production, and maintain bone health.

Development of Chronic Kidney Disease:

CKD typically develops slowly over months to years, often without noticeable symptoms in the early stages.

Common causes of CKD include diabetes, hypertension (high blood pressure), glomerulonephritis (inflammation of the kidney's filtering units), polycystic kidney disease (a genetic disorder causing cysts to form in the kidneys), and other conditions that impair kidney function.

As CKD progresses, the kidneys become less effective at filtering waste and maintaining fluid and electrolyte balance. This can lead to a buildup of waste products and fluid in the body, causing various symptoms and complications.

Stages of Chronic Kidney Disease:

CKD is categorized into five stages based on the estimated glomerular filtration rate (eGFR), a measure of how well the kidneys are filtering blood. These stages range from mild (stage 1) to severe (stage 5) kidney impairment.

Each stage is associated with specific symptoms, complications, and treatment approaches. For example, there may be no symptoms in the early stages, but as CKD progresses, symptoms such as fatigue, swelling, changes in urine output, and difficulty concentrating may develop.

Complications of Chronic Kidney Disease:

CKD can lead to various complications, including high blood pressure, fluid retention (edema), electrolyte imbalances, anemia, bone disease, cardiovascular disease, and kidney failure (end-stage renal disease, or ESRD).

Individuals with CKD are also at increased risk of developing other health problems, such as cardiovascular disease and infections, due to the compromised immune function associated with kidney dysfunction.

Management and Treatment:

Management of CKD aims to slow its progression, alleviate symptoms, and reduce the risk of complications.

Treatment may involve lifestyle modifications (such as dietary changes, exercise, and smoking cessation), medication to control blood pressure and manage symptoms, and, in advanced stages, renal replacement therapy (dialysis or kidney transplantation).

Basics: key nutrients to monitor in the renal diet

The basics of a renal diet revolve around managing the intake of certain nutrients to support kidney health and manage conditions like chronic kidney disease (CKD), kidney stones, and kidney failure. Here are some key principles of a renal diet:

Limit Sodium: High sodium intake can lead to fluid retention and high blood pressure, which can strain the kidneys. To reduce sodium intake, limit the use of table salt and avoid high-sodium processed foods such as canned soups, deli meats, and salty snacks.

Control Potassium: The kidneys play a key role in regulating potassium levels in the body. In individuals with kidney issues, high potassium levels can disrupt heart rhythm and muscle function. To control potassium intake, limit or avoid potassium-rich foods such as bananas, oranges, potatoes, tomatoes, and dairy products.

Manage Phosphorus: Excess phosphorus can contribute to bone and cardiovascular problems in people with kidney disease. To manage phosphorus intake, limit or avoid phosphorus-rich foods such as dairy products, nuts, seeds, chocolate, and certain processed foods.

Moderate Protein: While protein is essential for overall health, excessive protein intake can strain the kidneys. Individuals with kidney issues may benefit from moderating their protein intake while still ensuring adequate intake for muscle maintenance and repair. Lean protein sources such as poultry, fish, and eggs are often recommended.

Monitor Fluid Intake: Impaired kidney function can lead to difficulty regulating fluid levels in the body, resulting in fluid retention and swelling. To manage fluid intake, individuals with kidney issues may need to limit their fluid intake and monitor their fluid balance closely.

Individualized Approach: The renal diet is not one-size-fits-all; it should be tailored to each individual's specific kidney function, nutritional status, and other health conditions. Dietitians and healthcare providers work closely with patients to create personalized meal plans that meet their needs and preferences.

Focus on Nutrient-Rich Foods: Despite the restrictions, it's important to focus on consuming nutrient-rich foods that support overall health. This includes fruits, vegetables, whole grains, and lean proteins. These foods provide essential vitamins, minerals, and antioxidants that can help support kidney health and overall well-being.

Tips for managing fluid intake

Managing fluid intake is crucial for renal patients to help maintain fluid balance and prevent complications such as fluid overload and electrolyte imbalances. Here are some tips for managing fluid intake:

Monitor Fluid Intake: Keep track of your fluid intake throughout the day. This includes not only beverages but also foods with high water content, such as soups, fruits, and vegetables.

Limit Fluids: Follow your healthcare provider's recommendations regarding daily fluid intake limits. This limit may vary depending on your individual needs and stage of kidney disease.

Choose Fluids Wisely: Opt for beverages that are lower in sodium, potassium, and phosphorus. Examples include water, herbal teas, and small amounts of clear sodas. Avoid or limit high-sodium drinks like sports drinks, regular sodas, and some fruit juices.

Use Measuring Tools: Use measuring cups or a water bottle with measurements to track your fluid intake accurately.

Be Mindful of Thirst Triggers: Avoid salty or spicy foods, as they can increase thirst. Rinse canned vegetables and beans to reduce sodium content.

Limit Fluids at Mealtime: Try to drink most of your fluids between meals rather than during meals to prevent feeling overly full and to avoid diluting stomach acid, which aids in digestion.

Practice Portion Control: Use smaller glasses or cups to limit the amount of fluid consumed at one time. Sipping fluids slowly rather than drinking large amounts at once can help you feel satisfied with less.

Manage Thirst Sensations: Rinse your mouth with water or suck on ice chips if you feel thirsty between meals.

Monitor Urine Output: Pay attention to your urine output. Changes in urine volume or frequency may indicate fluctuations in fluid balance.

Consult with a Dietitian: Work with a registered dietitian who specializes in kidney disease to develop a personalized fluid management plan tailored to your specific needs and dietary restrictions.

CHAPTER 2: SHOPPING AND MEAL PLANNING FOR SENIORS

Grocery shopping tips for renal-friendly foods

Grocery shopping can be a key part of managing a renal diet for seniors. Below are some tips to make the process easier and more effective:

Plan Ahead: Before heading to the store, make a list of the items you need based on your renal diet guidelines. This can help you stay focused and avoid purchasing unnecessary or unhealthy foods.

Read Labels: Take the time to read nutrition labels on packaged foods to check for sodium, potassium, and phosphorus content. Look for products labeled "low-sodium" or "no added salt" for lower sodium options.

Choose Fresh Foods: Opt for fresh fruits and vegetables whenever possible, as they tend to have lower sodium and potassium content compared to canned or processed varieties. However, be mindful of high-potassium fruits and vegetables and choose lower-potassium options.

Limit Processed Foods: Processed and pre-packaged foods often contain high amounts of sodium, phosphorus, and other additives. Try to limit your intake of these items and focus on whole, minimally processed foods.

Shop the Perimeter: The perimeter of the grocery store typically contains fresh produce, lean meats, dairy, and other whole foods. Spend most of your time shopping in these areas to fill your cart with kidney-friendly options.

Stock Up on Staples: Keep your pantry stocked with kidney-friendly staples such as low-sodium broths, whole grains like rice and quinoa, and canned beans with no added salt.

Choose Lean Proteins: Select lean protein sources such as skinless poultry, fish, and tofu, which are lower in phosphorus and saturated fat compared to red meats.

Consider Convenience Foods: Look for convenient options like pre-cut fruits and vegetables or frozen meals labeled as kidney-friendly. Just be sure to check the nutrition label for sodium and potassium content.

Stay hydrated: Remember to drink plenty of water while you shop to stay hydrated, especially if you're following fluid restrictions as part of your renal diet.

Ask for Help: If you're unsure about certain foods or ingredients, don't hesitate to ask a store employee for assistance. Many stores also offer dietitian services or have resources available for customers with specific dietary needs.

Meal planning strategies for seniors with CKD

Meal planning for seniors with chronic kidney disease (CKD) involves careful consideration of nutrient intake to support kidney function while also addressing other health concerns common in older adults. Here are some meal-planning strategies tailored for seniors with CKD:

Consult a Dietitian: Work with a registered dietitian who specializes in kidney disease to create a personalized meal plan tailored to your individual needs, stage of CKD, and other health conditions.

Monitor Portion Sizes: Pay attention to portion sizes to avoid overeating, which can strain the kidneys. Use measuring cups or a food scale to ensure accuracy.

Focus on Fresh, Whole Foods: Prioritize fresh fruits and vegetables, lean proteins, and whole grains in your diet. These foods are typically lower in sodium, potassium, and phosphorus compared to processed options.

Limit Sodium Intake: Reduce your sodium intake by choosing fresh or frozen foods over canned and processed options. Use herbs, spices, and citrus juices to season foods instead of salt.

Manage Potassium and Phosphorus: Be mindful of foods high in potassium and phosphorus, as these minerals can build up in the blood in CKD. Choose lower-potassium fruits and vegetables and limit high-phosphorus foods like dairy, nuts, seeds, and processed meats.

Choose Lean Proteins: Opt for lean protein sources such as skinless poultry, fish, tofu, and egg whites, which are lower in phosphorus and saturated fat than red meats.

Include High-Quality Protein: Adequate protein intake is essential for seniors, but too much protein can strain the kidneys. Choose high-quality protein sources and spread your protein intake evenly throughout the day.

Monitor Fluid Intake: Follow your healthcare provider's recommendations for fluid intake, especially if you're on fluid restrictions. Limiting fluids can help manage fluid buildup and maintain electrolyte balance.

Plan Balanced Meals: Aim for balanced meals that include a variety of nutrient-rich foods from all food groups, including fruits, vegetables, whole grains, lean proteins, and healthy fats.

Stay Hydrated: Drink water throughout the day to stay hydrated, but be mindful of fluid restrictions if applicable. Monitor urine output and adjust fluid intake accordingly.

Limit Processed and Fast Foods: Minimize your intake of processed and fast foods, which are often high in sodium, phosphorus, and unhealthy fats. Cook meals at home whenever possible to have more control over ingredients.

Be Flexible: Don't be afraid to experiment with new recipes and ingredients to keep meals interesting and enjoyable. Focus on variety and moderation to meet your nutritional needs while managing CKD.

Budget-Friendly Renal Diet Options

Maintaining a renal diet on a budget is possible with some strategic planning and smart shopping. Here are some budget-friendly renal diet options for seniors:

Beans and Legumes: Beans and legumes like black beans, kidney beans, lentils, and chickpeas are affordable plant-based protein sources. They are also low in phosphorus and can be used in various dishes such as soups, salads, and stews.

Whole Grains: Choose budget-friendly whole grains such as brown rice, quinoa, barley, and oats. These grains are lower in phosphorus compared to refined grains and can be used as a base for meals or added to soups and salads.

Frozen Vegetables: Opt for frozen vegetables when fresh options are expensive or unavailable. Frozen vegetables are convenient, often cheaper than fresh produce, and retain their nutrients well. Choose low-potassium options such as green beans, cauliflower, and bell peppers.

Seasonal Fruits: Purchase seasonal fruits to save money and enjoy fresh produce at its peak. Choose lower-potassium options such as apples, berries, and grapes. Consider buying in bulk and freezing extra fruit for later use.

Eggs: Eggs are an inexpensive source of high-quality protein and can be incorporated into various dishes such as omelets, frittatas, and egg salads. They are also versatile and easy to prepare.

Canned Fish: Canned fish such as tuna, salmon, and sardines are budget-friendly sources of protein and omega-3 fatty acids. Look for varieties canned in water rather than oil to reduce sodium intake.

Low-Sodium Broths and Stocks: Use low-sodium broths and stocks as a base for soups, stews, and sauces. They add flavor to dishes without significantly increasing sodium intake.

Plant-based Proteins: Incorporate more plant-based proteins into your diet, such as tofu, tempeh, and seitan. These options are often cheaper than meat and poultry and can be used in place of animal proteins in many recipes.

Bulk Purchases: Buy pantry staples such as dried beans, rice, oats, and spices in bulk to save money in the long run. Look for sales and discounts on these items to maximize savings.

Meal Planning: Plan your meals to minimize food waste and make the most of ingredients you already have on hand. Use leftovers creatively to create new dishes and reduce the need for additional grocery shopping.

Grocery shopping list for renal diet

Protein Sources:

Skinless chicken breast

Lean cuts of beef or pork

Turkey

Fish (salmon, trout, tuna, and tilapia)

Shellfish (shrimp, crab, lobster)

Eggs

Low-sodium canned tuna or salmon

Tofu

Fruits and Vegetables:

Apples

Berries (strawberries, blueberries, raspberries)

Grapes

Pineapple

Peaches

Plums

Watermelon

Bell peppers (red, yellow, and green)

Cucumber

Cauliflower

Broccoli

Spinach

Kale

Zucchini

Carrots

Green beans

Eggplant

Radishes

Onions

Garlic

Tomatoes (in moderation due to potassium content)

Lettuce (romaine, iceberg)

Grains and Starches: (whole)

White rice (in moderation)

White bread (in moderation)

Pasta (in moderation)

Quinoa

Brown rice

Bulgur

Oats

Barley

Corn tortillas

Crackers (graham)

Dairy and Alternatives:

Low-fat or fat-free milk

Low-fat or fat-free yogurt

Low-fat or fat-free cheese

Cottage cheese

Unsweetened almond milk or soy milk

Dairy-free yogurt alternatives (made from almond, coconut, or soy)

Beans and Legumes:

Kidney beans

Black beans

Lentils

Chickpeas

Navy beans

Pinto beans

Condiments and Flavorings:

Herbs and spices (avoiding salt)

Olive oil or canola oil

Balsamic vinegar

Apple cider vinegar

Lemon juice

Low-sodium soy sauce or tamari

Mustard

Garlic powder

Onion powder

Maple syrups

Honey

Snacks and Beverages:

Unsalted nuts (almonds, cashews, walnuts)

Seeds (sunflower seeds, pumpkin seeds)

Popcorn (plain, unsalted)

Rice cakes

Low-sodium crackers

Fresh fruit juices (limit intake due to potassium content)

Herbal teas (caffeine-free)

Sparkling water

Vegetable Omelets

Ingredients

2 eggs

¼ cup chopped bell peppers

¼ cup chopped spinach

1 tbsp. olive oil

 Pepper to taste

Spring onion

½ onion diced

1 garlic cloves minced {optional}

Procedure

- Crack the eggs into a bowl and whisk until well combined, stir in onion and garlic if using.
- Stir in the chopped bell peppers, spring onion, and spinach.
- Heat olive oil in a non-stick frying pan over medium heat.
- Pour the egg mixture into the skillet and cook for 2-3 minutes until the bottom sets.
- Use a spatula to gently lift the edges of the omelet and allow the uncooked egg to flow underneath.
- Once the omelet is mostly set, fold it in half and cook for another 1-2 minutes until fully cooked.

Quinoa Porridge
Ingredients:

½ cup quinoa

1 cup almond milk

¼ tsp. cinnamon

¼ cup sliced strawberries

1 tbsp. honey

Procedure

- Rinse the quinoa under cold water.
- In a saucepan, combine the rinsed quinoa, almond milk, and cinnamon.
- Bring the mixture to a boil, then reduce the heat to low, cover, and simmer for about 15 minutes or until the quinoa is cooked and most liquid is absorbed.
- Stir and garnish with sliced strawberries and honey. Divide the porridge into bowls and serve warm.

Buckwheat Pancakes
Ingredients:

½ cup buckwheat flour

¼ cup almond milk

1 egg

¼ tsp. baking powder

1 tbsp. maple syrup

Procedure

- In a mixing bowl, combine the buckwheat flour, almond milk, egg, baking powder, and maple syrup. Whisk until smooth.
- Heat a non-stick skillet over medium heat and lightly grease with oil or cooking spray.
- Pour about ¼ cup of batter onto the skillet for each pancake.
- Cook for about 2-3 minutes until bubbles form on the surface, then flip and cook the other surface until golden brown.
- Repeat with the remaining batter.
- Serve warm with additional maple syrup if desired.

Almond Butter Toast
Ingredients:

2 slices whole grain bread

2 tbsp. almond butter

½ banana (sliced)

1 tsp. honey

Procedure

- Toast the two slices of whole-grain bread until golden brown.
- Spread 1 tablespoon of almond butter on each slice.

- Top with sliced banana. Drizzle with honey and serve

Smoothie Bowl
Ingredients:

½ cup frozen berries

½ banana

½ cup spinach

¼ cup almond milk

1 tbsp. chia seeds

Procedure

- In a blender, combine the frozen berries, banana, spinach, and almond milk.
- Blend until smooth and creamy. Pour the smoothie into a bowl.
- Top with chia seeds and additional berries if desired. Serve immediately with a spoon.

Egg Muffins
Ingredients:

4 eggs

¼ cup diced ham {pork}

¼ cup diced bell peppers {red, yellow, green}

Pepper to taste

Poultry seasoning to taste

Garlic powder {pinch}

1 tablespoon milk or milk substitute

½ cup onion

Salt (optional)

Procedure

- Grease a muffin tin and preheat oven to 350°F (175°C)
- Season the ham with garlic and seasonings, stir fry for some minutes (optional method)
- In a bowl, whisk the eggs and milk, then stir in the diced ham, onion, and bell peppers.
- Season with salt and pepper. Pour the egg mixture into the prepared muffin tin, filling each cup about 2/3 full.
- Bake for 15-20 minutes until the egg muffins are set and lightly golden. Allow to cool slightly before removing from the tin to a plate.

Cottage Cheese with Fruit
Ingredients:

½ cup cottage cheese

¼ cup pineapple chunks

¼ cup mandarin oranges

A pinch of cinnamon (optional)

Berries for toppings (optional)

Procedure

- In a bowl, combine the cottage cheese, pineapple chunks, and mandarin oranges.
- Mix well and sprinkle cinnamon if using. Serve chilled topped with berries if desired.

Rice Pudding
Ingredients:

½ cup cooked white rice

½ cup almond milk

¼ tsp. vanilla extract

1 tbsp. raisins

Procedure

- In a saucepan, combine the cooked white rice, almond milk, and vanilla extract.
- Cook over medium heat, stirring frequently, until the mixture thickens, about 10-15 minutes. Stir in the raisins.

Spinach and Feta Frittata
Ingredients:

4 eggs

½ cup chopped spinach

¼ cup crumbled feta cheese

Salt to taste

Black pepper to taste

½ teaspoon extra virgin oil

Procedure

- Preheat the oven to 350°F (175°C).
- In a bowl, whisk together the eggs, chopped spinach, and crumbled feta cheese—season with salt and pepper.
- Pour the mixture into a greased oven-safe skillet. Bake for 15-20 minutes until the frittata is set and golden brown on top. Slice and serve warm.

Or

On the skillet, fry the spinach for a few minutes or until wilted turning occasionally add the egg mixture (Egg, salt, pepper) to the pan, sprinkle with cheese, and transfer to the oven to bake for about 10 minutes.

Chia Seed Pudding
Ingredients:

2 tbsp. chia seeds

½ cup almond milk

¼ tsp. vanilla extract

1 tbsp. honey

Berries for toppings (optional)

Procedure

- In a bowl, whisk together the chia seeds, almond milk, vanilla extract, and honey.
- Cover and refrigerate for at least 2 hours or overnight, until the mixture thickens into a pudding-like consistency.
- Stir well before serving and top with berries if desired.

Whole Grain Waffles

Ingredients:

½ cup whole grain flour

½ cup almond milk

1 egg

¼ tsp. baking powder

1 tbsp. honey

½ tsp. vanilla extract

Toppings of choice

Procedure

- In a bowl, whisk together the whole-grain flour, almond milk, egg, baking powder, and honey until smooth.
- Preheat a waffle iron and lightly coat with cooking spray.
- Pour the batter onto the hot waffle iron and cook according to the manufacturer's instructions,

until golden brown and crisp. Serve warm with your choice of toppings.

Scrambled Tofu

Ingredients:

½ block tofu, crumbled

¼ cup diced tomatoes

¼ cup diced onions

¼ tsp. turmeric

2 tbsp. Bell peppers diced

Cauliflower/ spinach (optional)

A pinch of Salt (optional)

Black pepper to taste

½ tbsp. olive oil

Procedure

- Heat a skillet over medium heat and add the vegetables and stir, add the crumbled tofu. Cook for 2-3 minutes, stirring occasionally, until lightly browned.
- Add the diced tomatoes and onions to the skillet and cook for another 2-3 minutes until softened. Sprinkle turmeric over the mixture and stir to combine—season with salt and pepper to taste. Cook for an additional 1-2 minutes until heated through.

Mediterranean Breakfast Bowl

Ingredients:

½ cup cooked quinoa

¼ cup diced cucumber

¼ cup diced tomatoes

2 tbsp. crumbled feta cheese

1 tbsp. chopped fresh parsley

1 tbsp. lemon juice

Salt and pepper to taste

Procedure

- In a bowl, combine cooked quinoa, diced cucumber, diced tomatoes, crumbled feta cheese, and chopped fresh parsley.
- Drizzle with lemon juice and sprinkle with salt and pepper. Toss gently to combine. Serve immediately as a refreshing and nutritious breakfast option

Chia Seed Pancakes

Ingredients:

½ cup all-purpose flour

¼ cup chia seeds

1 tsp. baking powder

½ cup almond milk

1 egg

1 tbsp. honey

½ tsp. vanilla extract

Procedure

- In a mixing bowl, combine flour, chia seeds, and baking powder.
- In a separate bowl, whisk together almond milk, egg, honey, and vanilla extract.
- Combine wet ingredients with dry ingredients and mix until smooth.
- Grease the skillet with oil or butter and place over medium heat. Pour about ¼ cup of batter onto the skillet for each pancake.
- Cook for about 2-3 minutes until bubbles form on the surface, then flip and cook the other side for another 1-2 minutes until golden brown.
- Repeat with the remaining batter. Serve warm with your favorite toppings.

Sweet Potato Breakfast Hash
Ingredients:

1 medium sweet potato, diced

¼ cup diced bell peppers

¼ cup diced onions

¼ tsp. paprika

Salt (optional)

Pepper to taste (sprinkle)

1 tbsp. olive oil

Procedure

- Over medium heat, heat olive oil in a skillet.
- Add diced sweet potatoes and cook until they begin to soften, about 5-7 minutes. Add diced bell peppers, onions, paprika, salt, and pepper.
- Cook, stirring occasionally, until vegetables are tender and slightly browned, about 8-10 minutes.

Cauliflower Hash Browns
Ingredients:

1 cup grated cauliflower

1 egg

¼ cup grated cheese (optional)

½ onion diced

Salt and pepper to taste

Procedure

- In a mixing bowl, combine the grated cauliflower, onion, egg, and grated cheese (if using)—season with salt and pepper.
- Coat the skillet with cooking spray or oil over medium heat. Scoop about ¼ cup of the cauliflower mixture onto the skillet and flatten it into a round shape to form a hash brown.

- Cook for 3-4 minutes on each side until golden brown and crispy. Repeat with the remaining cauliflower mixture.

Cinnamon Raisin Toast
Ingredients:

2 slices whole grain bread

1 tbsp. almond butter

½ tsp. cinnamon

1 tbsp. raisins

Procedure

- Toast the slices of whole grain bread until crisps. Spread 1 tablespoon of almond butter evenly over each slice of toast. Sprinkle cinnamon over the almond butter. Top with raisins.

Egg White Vegetable Scramble
Ingredients:

4 egg whites

¼ cup diced bell peppers

¼ cup diced onions

¼ cup chopped spinach

¼ cup chopped mushroom/cauliflower

Spring onion for garnish

Salt to taste

Black pepper to taste

1 tsp. olive oil

Procedure

- In a non-stick skillet over medium heat, heat the olive oil. Add mushroom, diced bell peppers, and onions to the skillet and sauté until softened, about 3-4 minutes.
- Add chopped spinach to the skillet and cook until wilted, about 1-2 minutes. Pour egg whites into the skillet and season with salt and pepper.
- Cook, stirring occasionally, until the eggs are set and cooked through.
- Transfer to a plate and garnish with spring onion if desired.

Banana Nut Overnight Oats
Ingredients:

½ cup rolled oats

½ cup almond milk

½ ripe banana, mashed

1 tbsp. chopped nuts (such as almonds, walnuts, or pecans)

½ tsp. vanilla extract

½ tsp. cinnamon

1 tsp. Honey (optional)

Procedure

- In a jar or bowl, combine rolled oats, almond milk, mashed banana, chopped nuts, vanilla extract, and cinnamon. Stir well to combine all ingredients.
- Refrigerate for about four hours or overnight. In the morning, give the oats a good stir and add honey if desired for sweetness. Enjoy cold or heat in the microwave before serving.

Vegetable Breakfast Burrito

Ingredients:

2 large eggs, scrambled

¼ cup black beans, rinsed and drained

2 tbsp. diced bell peppers

2 tbsp. diced onions

2 tbsp. diced tomatoes

2 tbsp. shredded cheese

2 whole grain tortillas

½ tsp. ground cumin

Salt and pepper to taste

Procedure

- In a skillet over medium heat, sauté the diced bell peppers and onions until softened. Add the scrambled eggs to the skillet and cook until just set.

- Warm the black beans in the microwave or on the stovetop.
- Heat the tortillas in a skillet or microwave until warm and pliable.
- Divide the scrambled eggs, black beans, diced tomatoes, and shredded cheese between the two tortillas.
- Season with salt, cumin, and pepper to taste. Fold in the sides of each tortilla and roll tightly to form a burrito. Serve immediately, or wrap in foil for an on-the-go breakfast.

Blueberry Chia Seed Muffins
Ingredients:

1 cup all-purpose flour

½ cup almond milk

¼ cup maple syrup

¼ cup chia seeds

¼ cup coconut oil, melted

1 tsp. baking powder

½ tsp. vanilla extract

½ cup blueberries (fresh or frozen)

Procedure

- Preheat the oven to 350°F (175°C) and line a muffin tin with paper liners.
- In a mixing bowl, whisk together the almond milk, maple syrup, melted coconut oil, and vanilla extract.
- In a separate bowl, combine the flour, chia seeds, and baking powder.
- Gently add the dry and wet ingredients, stirring until just well combined. Gently fold in the blueberries.
- Divide the batter evenly among the muffin cups. Bake for about 20-25 minutes, or until a toothpick or tester inserted into the center of the muffin comes out clean.
- Give it time to cool in the muffins before transferring to a wire rack to cool completely

Mushroom and Spinach Breakfast Quesadilla

Ingredients:

2 whole grain tortillas

½ cup sliced mushrooms

1 cup fresh spinach leaves

¼ cup shredded cheese

2 tbsp. salsa (optional)

Cooking spray

Salt and pepper to taste

Procedure

- Heat a non-stick skillet over medium heat and lightly coat with cooking spray.
- Add the sliced mushrooms to the skillet and cook until softened about 3-4 minutes. Add the fresh spinach leaves to the skillet and cook until wilted, about 1-2 minutes.
- Season with salt and pepper to taste. Remove the mushrooms and spinach from the skillet and set aside.
- Place one tortilla in the skillet and sprinkle half of the shredded cheese evenly over the surface.
- Top with the cooked mushrooms and spinach, followed by the remaining shredded cheese.
- Place the second tortilla on top of the filled one and press down gently.
- Cook for 2-3 minutes on each side, or until the quesadilla is golden brown and the cheese is melted.
- Slice into wedges and serve hot, with salsa if desired.

Eggplant Parmesan

Ingredients: 2 servings

1 large eggplant, sliced into rounds

½ cup whole wheat breadcrumbs

¼ cup grated Parmesan cheese

2 eggs, beaten

1 cup marinara sauce (store-bought or homemade)

½ cup shredded mozzarella cheese

1 tbsp. chopped fresh basil (for garnish, optional)

Procedure

- Preheat the oven to 375°F (190°C). Dip eggplant slices in beaten eggs, then coat with a mixture of whole wheat breadcrumbs and grated Parmesan cheese.
- Place coated eggplant slices on a baking sheet lined with parchment paper.
- Bake for about 20-25 minutes or until golden brown and crispy.
- Spread marinara sauce evenly in the bottom of a baking dish. Place baked eggplant slices on top of the sauce. Top with shredded mozzarella cheese.
- Return to the oven and bake for another 15-20 minutes, or until the cheese is melted and bubbly. Garnish with chopped fresh basil before serving if desired.

Turkey and Black Bean Tacos

Ingredients: 2 servings

4 whole grain tortillas

½ lb. ground turkey

½ cup canned black beans drained and rinsed

¼ cup diced onions

¼ cup diced bell peppers

1 clove garlic, minced

½ tsp. chili powder

½ tsp. ground cumin

Salt and pepper to taste

¼ cup salsa (optional)

¼ cup shredded lettuce (for garnish, optional)

¼ cup diced tomatoes (for garnish, optional)

Procedure

- Over medium heat, heat olive oil in a skillet. Add minced garlic, diced onions, and diced bell peppers. Cook until softened, about 3-4 minutes.
- Add ground turkey to the skillet, breaking each part with a spoon and stirring, cook until browned.
- Add canned black beans, chili powder, ground cumin, salt, and pepper to the skillet. Cook for another 2-3 minutes to heat through.

- Warm whole-grain tortillas in a dry skillet or microwave. Spoon turkey and black bean mixture onto each tortilla. Top with salsa, shredded lettuce, and diced tomatoes if desired.

Pesto Pasta Salad with Cherry Tomatoes

Ingredients: 2 servings

1 cup cooked whole grain pasta

½ cup cherry tomatoes, halved

2 tbsp. prepared pesto sauce

1 tbsp. olive oil

1 tbsp. balsamic vinegar

Salt and pepper to taste

1 tbsp. chopped fresh basil (for garnish, optional)

Procedure

- In a bowl, combine cooked whole-grain pasta and cherry tomatoes.
- In a small bowl, whisk together prepared pesto sauce, olive oil, and balsamic vinegar. Pour pesto dressing over the pasta and tomatoes. Toss to coat evenly.
- Season with salt and pepper to taste. Garnish with chopped fresh basil before serving if desired.

Mushroom and Spinach Quiche
Ingredients: 4 servings

1 whole grain pie crust (store-bought or homemade)

4 large eggs

½ cup milk (or unsweetened almond milk)

½ cup sliced mushrooms

1 cup chopped fresh spinach leaves

¼ cup diced onions

2 garlic cloves minced

½ tbsp. Dijon mustard (optional)

¼ tsp., thyme

½ cup low-fat shredded cheese (such as Swiss or Gruyere)

Salt and pepper to taste

Procedure

- Preheat the oven to 375°F (190°C). Line a pie dish with the whole grain pie crust.
- In a bowl, whisk together eggs and milk—season with salt and pepper.
- In a skillet, heat olive oil over medium heat. Add sliced mushrooms, diced onions, garlic, thyme, Mustard, and fresh spinach leaves. Cook until vegetables are tender and wilted.
- Spread cooked vegetables evenly over the bottom of the pie crust. Sprinkle shredded cheese on top.

- Pour the egg mixture over the vegetables and cheese in the pie crust. Bake in the preheated oven for 30-35 minutes, or until the quiche is set and golden brown on top. Allow to cool slightly before serving.

Shrimp and Vegetable Skewers

Ingredients: 2 servings

8 large shrimp, peeled and deveined

½ cup cherry tomatoes

½ cup bell pepper chunks

½ cup zucchini chunks

½ onion chunks

1 tbsp. olive oil

1 clove garlic, minced

1 tsp. Smoked paprika

½ tsp. cumin

Salt and pepper to taste

Procedure

- Preheat the grill or grill pan to medium heat. In a bowl, toss shrimp, cherry tomatoes, bell pepper chunks, and zucchini chunks with olive oil, minced garlic, paprika, cumin, salt, and pepper.

- Thread shrimp and vegetables onto skewers, alternating as desired. Grill skewers for 2-3 minutes on each side, or until shrimp are pink and cooked through and vegetables are tender. garnish with fresh parsley or dill if desired

Vegetable and Tofu Stir-Fry
Ingredients: 2 servings

½ block firm tofu, cubed

1 cup mixed vegetables (like bell peppers, snap peas, broccoli and carrots)

2 tbsp. low-sodium soy sauce

1 tbsp. hoisin sauce

1 clove garlic, minced

½ tsp. grated fresh ginger

1 tbsp. olive oil

½ tsp. cumin

Black pepper to taste

Sesame seeds for garnish (optional)

Procedure

- Heat olive oil in a wok or skillet over medium-high heat. Add minced garlic and grated fresh ginger to the skillet. Cook until fragrant, about 1 minute.

- Add cubed tofu to the skillet. Cook until golden brown on all sides. Add mixed vegetables to the skillet. Stir-fry until vegetables are tender-crisp. Add the pepper and cumin.
- In a small bowl, whisk together low-sodium soy sauce and hoisin sauce. Pour over the tofu and vegetables in the skillet. Stir to coat evenly and cook for another 2-3 minutes. Serve hot, garnished with sesame seeds if desired.
- Serve over cooked brown rice

Tuna Salad Stuffed with Bell Peppers
Ingredients: 2 servings

2 large bell peppers

1 can (5 oz.) tuna in water, drained

¼ cup diced celery

¼ cup diced red onion

2 tbsp. plain Greek yogurt

1 tbsp. lemon juice

Salt and black pepper to taste

½ tbsp. cumin

1 garlic clove minced

½ cup shredded low-fat cheese (optional)

1 tbsp. chopped fresh parsley or dill (optional)

Procedure

- Preheat the oven to 350°F (175°C). Cut the bell peppers in half lengthwise and remove the seeds and membranes. In a bowl, mix drained tuna, diced celery, diced red onion, Greek yogurt, lemon juice, cumin, garlic, salt, and pepper.
- Stuff each bell pepper half with the tuna salad mixture and spread cheese on top if using. Place stuffed bell peppers on a baking sheet and bake in the preheated oven for 15-20 minutes, or until the peppers are tender. Garnish with chopped fresh parsley if desired.

Mediterranean Chickpea Salad
Ingredients: 2 servings

1 can (15 oz.) chickpeas, rinsed and drained

½ cup diced cucumber

½ cup diced tomatoes

¼ cup diced red onion

¼ cup chopped fresh parsley

2 tbsp. chopped fresh mint

2 tbsp. crumbled feta cheese

1 tbsp. olive oil

1 tbsp. lemon juice

Salt and pepper to taste

Procedure

- In a large bowl, combine chickpeas, diced cucumber, diced tomatoes, diced red onion, chopped fresh parsley, chopped fresh mint, and crumbled feta cheese.
- Drizzle olive oil and lemon juice over the salad—season with salt and pepper. Toss to combine all ingredients. Serve chilled or at room temperature.

Caprese Stuffed Portobello Mushrooms

Ingredients: **2 servings**

2 large Portobello mushrooms

½ cup diced tomatoes

¼ cup sliced fresh mozzarella cheese

2 tbsp. chopped fresh basil

1 tbsp. balsamic glaze

1 small garlic clove minced

1 tsp. olive oil

Salt and pepper to taste

Procedure

- Preheat the oven to 400°F (200°C). Remove the stems from the Portobello mushrooms and carefully scrape out the gills, grease the mushroom with some oil mixed with pepper, salt, and garlic.

- In a bowl, combine diced tomatoes, sliced fresh mozzarella cheese, oil, chopped fresh basil, balsamic glaze, garlic, salt, and pepper. Stuff each Portobello mushroom with a tomato and mozzarella mixture.
- Place the filled mushrooms on a baking sheet lined with parchment paper. Bake in the preheated oven for 15-20 minutes, or until mushrooms are tender and cheese is melted and bubbly.

Turkey and Vegetable Skillet
Ingredients: **2 servings**

½ lb. ground turkey

½ cup diced bell peppers

½ cup diced zucchini

¼ cup diced onions

1 clove garlic, minced

Broccoli florets

½ tsp. Italian seasoning or mix of sage, oregano, basil, and rosemary blended.

Salt and pepper to taste

1 tbsp. olive oil

Procedure

- In a skillet over medium heat, heat the olive oil. Add the minced garlic and diced onions to the skillet. Cook for approximately 3-4 minutes, or until the onions are transparent.

- Add ground turkey to the skillet. Cook until browned and cooked through, breaking it apart with a spoon.
- Add diced bell peppers, broccoli, and diced zucchini to the skillet. Cook until vegetables are tender, about 5-7 minutes—season with Italian seasoning, salt, and pepper.

Quinoa Salad with Roasted Vegetables
Ingredients: 1 serving

½ cup cooked quinoa

1 cup mixed roasted vegetables (such as bell peppers, zucchini, broccoli and cherry tomatoes)

1 tbsp. olive oil

1 medium garlic clove minced

½ tsp. dried rosemary

Salt and black pepper to taste

1 tbsp. balsamic vinegar

Procedure

- Preheat the oven to 400°F (200°C). Toss mixed vegetables with olive oil, rosemary, garlic, salt, and pepper.
- Roast in the oven for about 20-25 minutes, or until tender. In a bowl, combine cooked quinoa

and roasted vegetables. Sprinkle with balsamic vinegar and toss to coat.

Chicken and Vegetable Soup
Ingredients: 2 servings

1 boneless, skinless chicken breast (4 oz.)

4 cups low-sodium chicken broth

1 cup mixed vegetables (such as carrots, celery, and onions)

½ cup cooked whole-grain pasta

Salt and pepper to taste

1 tbsp. chopped fresh parsley (optional)

NOTE: This recipe can also be enjoyed by using uncooked wide noodles and already-cooked rotisserie chicken

Procedure

- In a pot, bring chicken broth to a boil. Add chicken breast and mixed vegetables to the pot. Reduce heat and simmer for 15-20 minutes, or until chicken is cooked through.
- Remove the chicken from the pot, shred it with two forks, and return it to the pot. Add cooked pasta to the pot and season with salt and pepper. Serve hot, garnished with chopped fresh parsley if desired.

Greek Salad with Grilled Chicken

Ingredients:

4 oz. grilled chicken breast

2 cups mixed salad greens

¼ cup cucumber slices

¼ cup cherry tomatoes, halved

¼ avocado

¼ green pepper sliced

2 tbsp. crumbled feta cheese or cubed

1 tbsp. Kalamata olives

1 tbsp. olive oil

1 tbsp. balsamic vinegar

Salt to taste (optional)

Cracked pepper to taste

Procedure

- In a large bowl, combine mixed salad greens, cucumber slices, cherry tomatoes, crumbled feta cheese, and Kalamata olives.
- Drizzle olive oil and balsamic vinegar over the salad. Season with salt and pepper. Toss to coat evenly. Top with grilled chicken breast

Lemon Garlic Shrimp with Quinoa
Ingredients: 1 serving

8 large shrimp, peeled and deveined

½ cup cooked quinoa

1 tbsp. olive oil

1 clove garlic, minced

1 tbsp. lemon juice

½ tsp. lemon zest

Salt to taste

Cayenne pepper to taste

1 tbsp. chopped fresh parsley for garnish (optional)

Procedure

- Heat olive oil in a skillet over medium heat. Add minced garlic and stir until fragrant, about 1 minute.
- Add shrimp to the skillet and cook until pink and opaque, about 2-3 minutes per side.
- Season shrimp with lemon juice, lemon zest, salt, and pepper.
- Serve shrimp over cooked quinoa. Garnish with chopped fresh parsley if desired.

Note: you can make it more delightful by adding vegetables like zucchini, and carrots in the quinoa.

You can also alternate with chicken and orzo pasta adhering to renal-friendly recipes.

Vegetable and Lentil Soup
Ingredients: 4 servings

½ cup dried green lentils

4 cups low-sodium vegetable broth

1 cup mixed vegetables (such as carrots, celery, and onions)

½ cup diced tomatoes

1 clove garlic, minced

½ tsp. dried thyme (optional)

2 tablespoons lemon juice

½ tsp. dried rosemary

Salt and pepper to taste

1 tbsp. olive oil

1 tbsp. chopped fresh parsley for garnish

Procedure

- Rinse the green lentils under cold water and drain. In a pot, heat olive oil over medium heat. Add minced garlic and cook until fragrant, about 1 minute. Add mixed vegetables to the pot and cook until slightly softened about 5 minutes.
- Add dried green lentils, diced tomatoes, dried thyme, dried rosemary, and vegetable broth to the pot. Bring to a boil.
- Reduce heat and simmer for 20-25 minutes, or until lentils are tender—season with salt and

pepper to taste. Serve hot, garnished with chopped fresh parsley if desired.

Cauliflower Rice Stir-Fry
Ingredients: 4 servings

1 head cauliflower, grated into rice-like texture

1 cup chopped mixed vegetables (bell peppers, carrots, peas)

2 cloves garlic, minced

1 medium onion diced

½ cup purple cabbage (optional)

2 tablespoons low-sodium soy sauce

1 tablespoon sesame oil

2 stalks green onions or spring onion chopped

Salt and pepper to taste

Procedure

- Heat sesame oil in a skillet, add garlic, and onion, and stir for a minute.
- Add cauliflower rice and mixed vegetables. Cook until vegetables are tender.
- Add soy sauce, green onions, salt, and pepper, and mix well.

Chicken and Vegetable Lettuce Wraps

Ingredients: 2 servings

4 large lettuce leaves (such as romaine or iceberg)

4 oz. cooked chicken breast, shredded

½ cup shredded carrots

½ cup sliced cucumber

¼ cup diced red bell pepper

2 tbsp. chopped fresh cilantro

½ red onion diced

2 tbsp. hoisin sauce

1 tbsp. low-sodium soy sauce

1 tbsp. rice vinegar

1 tsp. sesame oil

Procedure

- In a small bowl, combine hoisin sauce, low-sodium soy sauce, rice vinegar, and sesame oil to make the sauce.
- Divide shredded chicken breast, shredded carrots, sliced cucumber, diced red bell pepper, and chopped fresh cilantro among the lettuce leaves. Drizzle sauce over the filling in each lettuce wrap.
- Serve immediately, folding the lettuce leaves over the filling to eat.

Mushroom and Spinach Frittata

Ingredients: 4-6 servings

8 eggs

1 cup sliced mushrooms

2 cups fresh spinach

1 teaspoon fresh dried dill

½ cup diced onion

½ cup shredded low-fat cheese

1 tablespoon olive oil

1 clove garlic minced

A pinch of thyme

¼ tablespoon black pepper

Procedure

- Preheat oven to 350°F (175°C), sauté onion and garlic in the olive oil for about 3- 5 minutes, add mushroom, thyme, and finally spinach.
- Whisk eggs in a bowl, and add sautéed vegetables, dill, pepper, and cheese. Stir in the sautéed mushroom-spinach mixture
- Pour the mixture into a greased baking dish and bake until the center of the frittata is firm. (about 20-25)

Rice Noodles with Vegetables

Ingredients: 6 servings

8 oz. rice noodles

1 tablespoon olive oil

2 cloves garlic, minced

1 cup sliced bell peppers (any color)

1 cup sliced carrots

1 cup sliced zucchini

1 cup sliced mushrooms

1 cup baby spinach leaves

2 tablespoons low-sodium soy sauce

1 tablespoon rice vinegar

1 teaspoon grated fresh ginger

Pepper to taste

Green onions for garnish

Sesame seeds for garnish (optional)

Procedure

- Cook and drain the rice noodles according to package instructions.
- On a medium heat, heat the olive oil in a skillet or wok. Add the minced garlic to the skillet and cook until fragrant. Add the sliced bell peppers, carrots, zucchini, and mushrooms to the skillet. Stir-fry for 5-7 minutes, or until the vegetables

are tender-crisp. Add the baby spinach leaves to the skillet and cook for an additional 1-2 minutes, until wilted.

- In a small bowl, whisk together the low-sodium soy sauce, rice vinegar, and grated fresh ginger. Pour the sauce over the vegetables in the skillet and toss to coat evenly. Cook for another 1-2 minutes.
- Gently add the noodles to the skillet and toss to combine thoroughly, cook for about 2-3 minutes to heat through. Taste and season with pepper as needed.
- Garnish with chopped green onions and sesame seeds, if desired.

Vegetable Stir-Fry
Ingredients: 2-3 servings

2 cups mixed vegetables (broccoli or mushroom, snap peas, celery)

2 tablespoons olive oil

2 cloves garlic, minced

1 medium red bell pepper

1 medium green bell pepper

4 cherry tomatoes (optional)

½ small onion

½ teaspoon dried oregano

¼ teaspoon ground pepper

1 tablespoon low-sodium soy sauce

Procedure

- Heat oil in a large skillet, add mushroom, celery bell peppers, oregano, onion, and snap peas until tender

- Add pepper, tomatoes, and soy sauce and stir

- Serve on brown rice or quinoa

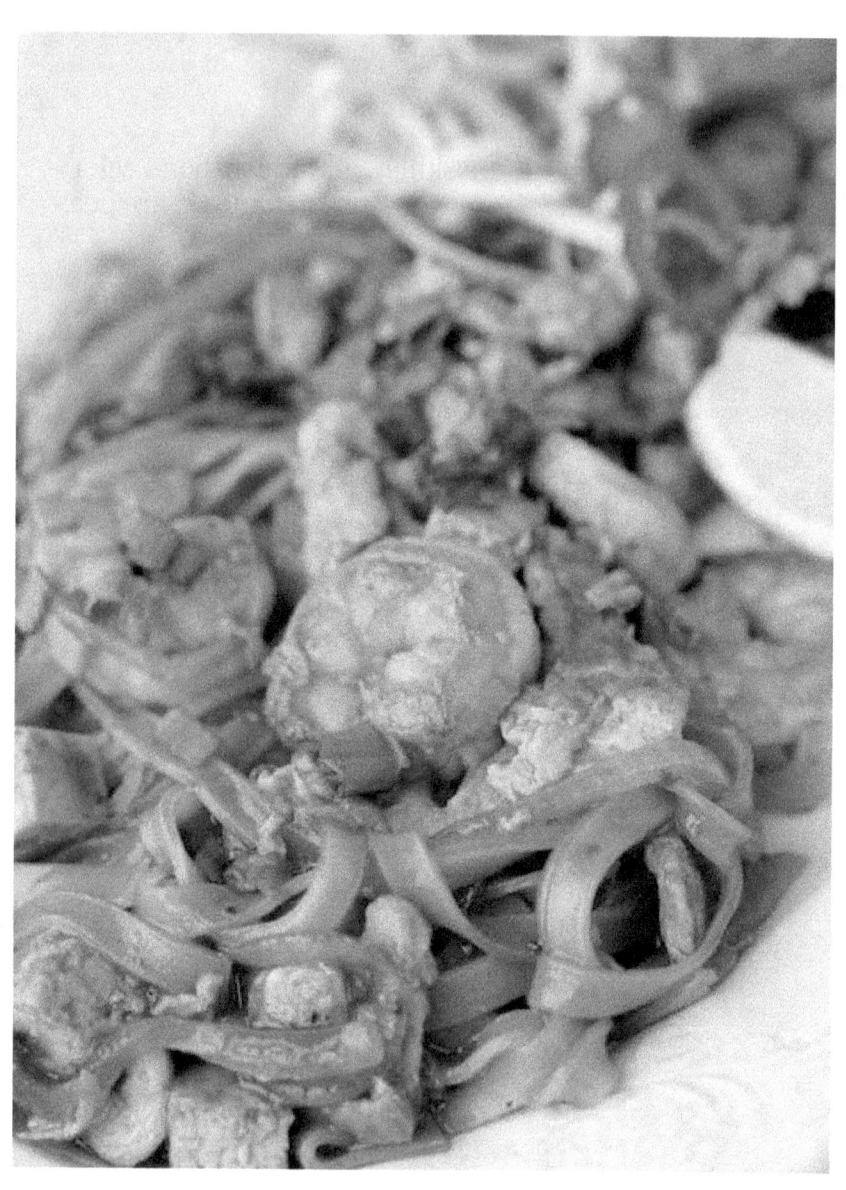

Baked Chicken Breast with Roasted Vegetables

Ingredients: 4 servings

4 boneless, skinless chicken breasts

2 tablespoons olive oil

1 teaspoon garlic powder

1 teaspoon paprika

½ teaspoon rosemary

Salt and pepper to taste

Assorted vegetables (zucchini, bell peppers, onions, broccoli, etc.)

Procedure

- Preheat the oven to 400°F (200°C). Rub chicken breasts with olive oil and season with garlic powder, rosemary, paprika, salt, and pepper.
- Place chicken breasts on a baking sheet lined with parchment paper.
- Toss assorted vegetables with olive oil, salt, and pepper. Arrange vegetables around the chicken on the baking sheet.
- Bake for 20-25 minutes or until chicken is cooked through and vegetables are tender.
- Serve chicken alongside roasted chicken.

Sweet Potato and Black Bean Quesadillas

Ingredients:

2 medium sweet potatoes, peeled and diced

1 can black beans, drained and rinsed

1 teaspoon chili powder

½ teaspoon cumin

½ teaspoon paprika

1 large bell pepper

4 whole wheat tortillas

Extra-virgin oil

1 cup shredded cheese (such as cheddar or Monterey Jack)

Guacamole and salsa for serving

Procedure

- Boil diced sweet potatoes until tender, about 10–15 minutes; drain and mash.
- In a bowl, mix mashed sweet potatoes, black beans, chili powder, paprika, and cumin.
- Heat a skillet over medium heat. Sauté onion, garlic, and bell pepper, and mix it in the potato bowl.
- Place a tortilla in the skillet and spread the sweet potato mixture evenly on one half. Sprinkle shredded cheese over the sweet potato mixture.

Fold the tortilla in half to cover the filling and press down gently.

- Cook until the bottom is golden brown, then flip and cook the other side until golden brown and crispy. Repeat with the remaining tortillas and filling.
- **Servings:** Serve quesadillas with guacamole or salsa, plain non-fat Greek yogurt, light sour cream, and diced avocado if desired.

Vegetarian Chili
Ingredients: 4-6 servings

1 can kidney beans, drained and rinsed

1 can black beans, drained and rinsed

1 can diced tomatoes

1 onion, diced

Celery

1 carrot diced

1 bell pepper, diced

2 cloves garlic, minced

2 tablespoons chili powder

1 teaspoon cumin

2 tablespoons dried oregano

Water/ vegetable broth for cooking

Procedure

- In a large pot, sauté the onion, bell pepper, and garlic until softened. Add kidney beans, black beans, diced tomatoes, chili powder, cumin, salt, oregano, carrot, celery and pepper.
- Bring to a simmer and cook for 20–25 minutes. Adjust the seasoning if necessary before serving.

Mushroom and Spinach Pasta

Ingredients:

8 oz. whole wheat pasta

2 cups sliced mushrooms

2 cups fresh spinach leaves

2 cloves garlic, minced

2 tablespoons olive oil

1 tablespoon balsamic vinegar

¼ cup grated Parmesan cheese

Pepper to taste

Procedure

- Cook pasta according to package instructions and drain—heat olive oil in a skillet over medium heat.
- Add garlic and mushrooms, and sauté until the mushrooms are tender. Stir in the spinach and cook until wilted.

- Sprinkle vinegar and toss cooked pasta with the mushroom and spinach mixture. Season with pepper, and sprinkle with Parmesan cheese before serving.

NOTE: This recipe can be made creamy by adding 1 cup of half-and-half creamer.

Black Bean and Sweet Potato Tacos
Ingredients:

1 can black beans, rinsed and drained

2 cups diced sweet potatoes

1 teaspoon chili powder

½ teaspoon cumin

¼ teaspoon paprika

Salt and pepper to taste

Corn tortillas

Toppings: avocado, salsa, cilantro, lime wedges

Procedure

- Preheat the oven to 400°F (200°C). Toss sweet potatoes with chili powder, cumin, paprika, salt, and pepper.
- Spread sweet potatoes on a baking sheet and roast for 20–25 minutes, or until tender.
- Heat black beans in a saucepan over medium heat.

- Warm corn tortillas. Assemble tacos with black beans, roasted sweet potatoes, and desired toppings.

Chicken and Vegetable Skewers

Ingredients: **4 servings**

1-pound boneless, skinless chicken thigh cut into chunks (turkey can also do)

1 tablespoon peach jam

2 bell peppers, cut into squares

1 zucchini, sliced

2 tablespoons olive oil

1 medium onion

1 medium yellow summer squash

1 teaspoon paprika

Pinch of dried ground sage

Salt and pepper to taste

Procedure

- Make the marinade by mixing the olive oil, peach jam, paprika, sage, salt, and pepper and stirring until blended.
- Add some marinade to the chicken and refrigerate to marinate.

- Place the already bite-sized vegetable in a bowl and add the reserved marinade, stir to coat the vegetables
- Preheat the grill or broiler and Thread chicken, bell peppers, onion, and zucchini onto skewers.
- Grill for 10-15 minutes covered and turn occasionally to cook evenly

Turkey Meatball Subs
Ingredients: 4 servings

1 lb. ground turkey (beef can also do)

½ cup breadcrumbs

1 egg

¼ cup grated Parmesan cheese

1 teaspoon Italian seasoning (dried leaves like thyme, rosemary, basil, oregano and more blended)

4 whole wheat sub rolls

1 cup marinara sauce

1 cup shredded mozzarella cheese

Procedure

- Preheat the oven to 375°F (190°C). In a bowl, mix ground turkey, breadcrumbs, eggs, Parmesan cheese, and Italian seasoning.
- Form the mixture into meatballs and place them on a baking sheet. Bake for about 20–25 minutes, or until cooked through.

- Heat the marinara sauce in a saucepan. Place cooked meatballs in sub rolls, and top with marinara sauce and mozzarella cheese. Bake subs for 5-10 minutes or until cheese is melted and bubbly.

Salmon and Vegetable Foil Packets

Ingredients:

4 salmon fillets

2 cups mixed vegetables (zucchini, bell peppers, onions, and asparagus)

4 tablespoons lemon juice

4 tablespoons olive oil

4 cloves garlic, minced or garlic powder

1 tablespoon smoked paprika

Fresh or dry oregano/ parsley

Salt and cayenne pepper to taste

Procedure

- Preheat the oven to 400°F (200°C). Place each salmon fillet on a large piece of foil. Divide the mixed vegetables among the foil packets.
- In a small bowl, mix lemon juice, olive oil, garlic, salt, paprika, oregano, and pepper. Drizzle over salmon and vegetables. Fold foil to seal packets.
- Bake for about 15-20 minutes or until salmon is cooked through and vegetables are tender.

Ratatouille

Ingredients: **4-7 servings**

1 eggplant, diced

2 zucchinis, diced

2 carrots diced

1 red bell pepper, diced

1 green bell pepper diced

2 tomatoes, diced

1 large onion, diced

3 cloves garlic, minced

2 tablespoons olive oil

1 tablespoon of fresh rosemary

1 tablespoon zest (optional)

1 tablespoon fresh basil

1 teaspoon dried thyme

8 tablespoons grated parmesan cheese (optional)

Ground black pepper to taste

Procedure

- Heat olive oil in a skillet over medium heat and add diced onion and garlic, cook until softened. Add diced eggplant, zucchini, bell peppers, zest if using, basil, rosemary, thyme, and pepper. Cook for 10-15 minutes or until tender stirring occasionally.

- Add the tomatoes and cheese if using and mix well, simmering covered until vegetables are ready. Serve hot as a side dish or add pasta, you can also add cooked ground turkey, chicken, or beef to make it whole.

Tilapia with Mango Salsa

Ingredients: **4 servings**

4 tilapia fillets

2 teaspoons paprika

1 teaspoon dried thyme

1 teaspoon onion powder

1 teaspoon garlic powder

½ teaspoon cayenne pepper

½ teaspoon black pepper

½ teaspoon salt

1 tablespoon fresh minced parsley

2 tablespoons olive oil

For Mango Salsa:

1 ripe mango, diced

½ red onion, finely chopped

¼ cup chopped fresh cilantro

Juice of 1 lime

Salt and pepper to taste

Procedure

- In a small bowl, mix paprika, thyme, onion powder, garlic powder, cayenne pepper, black pepper, parsley, lemon juice, and salt. Rub this spice mixture onto both sides of the tilapia fillets and refrigerate in a sealable bag to marinate for about an hour.
- Heat olive oil in a skillet. Cook the tilapia for 3-4 minutes on each side until the fish is blackened and cooked through.
- For the mango salsa, combine diced mango, chopped red onion, cilantro, lime juice, and salt in a bowl. Mix well and Serve the blackened tilapia topped with mango salsa.

Greek Yogurt Chicken Salad
Ingredients: 4 servings

2 cups cooked shredded chicken

½ cup diced celery

½ cup halved grapes

¼ cup chopped walnuts

½ cup Greek yogurt

¼ cup low-fat mayonnaise

2 tablespoons lemon juice

1 tablespoon fresh dill

1 tablespoon fresh parsley

1 tablespoon honey

Black pepper to taste

Iceberg Lettuce leaves for servings

Procedure

- Mix chicken, celery, grapes, fresh dill, parsley, and walnuts in a bowl. Stir in Greek yogurt, lemon juice, and pepper.
- Serve chilled as a sandwich filling or over lettuce leaves.

Chicken and Broccoli Alfredo
Ingredients: 4-5 servings

8 oz. whole wheat fettuccine pasta

2 boneless, skinless chicken breasts, cut into strips

2 cups broccoli florets

2 cloves garlic, minced

1 cup low-sodium chicken broth or lemon juice

1 cup low-fat milk or half-and-half creamer

¼ cup grated Parmesan cheese

1 teaspoon ground peppercorn

2 tablespoons olive oil

Red bell pepper for garnish (optional)

Pepper to taste

Procedure

- Cook pasta according to package instructions without salt add broccoli in the last minutes and drain.
- Heat olive oil in a pan over medium heat, add chicken strips and minced garlic, cook until browned.
- Pour in chicken broth, and milk, and bring to a boil Stir in cooked pasta, peppercorn, garlic powder, and grated Parmesan cheese. Cook for a few more minutes until the sauce thickens, sprinkle with pepper and bell pepper.

Veggie Lentil Burgers

Ingredients: 4 servings

1 cup cooked lentils

1 cup chopped mixed vegetables (bell peppers, carrots, onions)

½ cup breadcrumbs

1 egg

2 tablespoons olive oil

1 teaspoon paprika

½ teaspoon dried oregano

2 tablespoons walnuts chopped (optional)

¼ teaspoon garlic powder

Salt and pepper to taste

Procedure

- In a bowl, mash cooked lentils. Add chopped vegetables, breadcrumbs, egg, garlic, walnuts, paprika, salt, and pepper. Mix well.
- Form the mixture into burger patties, Heat olive oil in a skillet over medium heat. Cook the patties until each side turns golden brown and cooked.
- Serve in buns or lettuce wraps with your favorite toppings adhering to renal-friendly ingredients.

Roasted Vegetable Pasta (primavera)

Ingredients: **3 servings**

8 oz. whole wheat pasta

2 cups mixed roasted vegetables (bell peppers, cherry tomatoes, squash, carrot, and broccoli)

2 tablespoons olive oil

2 cloves garlic, minced

¼ cup grated Parmesan cheese

1 tablespoon of all-purpose flour

2 tablespoons half-and-half creamer (optional)

1 cup low-sodium chicken broth

Procedure

- Cook pasta according to package instructions without salt. Drain and set aside.

- Roast or cook the vegetables until tender

- In a pan, heat olive oil, add garlic, and sauté.

- Pour in the chicken stock and cook on low heat.

- Add the all-purpose flour and stir to avoid clumps, add half and half and simmer.

- Toss in roasted vegetables and cooked pasta. Sprinkle with Parmesan cheese.

Note: This recipe can be enjoyed without cream, stock, and, flour by:

- Frying your garlic with oil, add the pasta, and vegetables and cook, and finally adding the cheese

Chicken and Vegetable Brown Rice
Ingredients: **3 servings**

2 cups brown rice cooked

2 chicken breasts, cooked and shredded

1 ½ cup mixed vegetables (peas, carrots, corn, bell peppers, broccoli or mushroom)

1 clove minced garlic (optional)

½ onion cut into small wedges

2 tablespoons low-sodium soy sauce

1 tablespoon sesame oil

Procedure

- In a pan, combine cooked brown rice, shredded chicken, and mixed vegetables. Stir in soy sauce and sesame oil. Cook for 5-7 minutes until heated through.

OR

- Sauté onion, and garlic in oil, add the shredded chicken, vegetables, and soy sauce, and serve over the cooked brown rice

Spaghetti Squash with Tomato Sauce
Ingredients: 4 servings

1 medium spaghetti squash

2 cups low-sodium tomato sauce

1 teaspoon dried basil

1 medium shallot diced

1 teaspoon dried oregano

2 cloves garlic, minced

2 tablespoons olive oil

Pepper to taste

Procedure

- Preheat oven to 400°F. Cut spaghetti squash in half lengthwise, scoop out seeds, and place face down on a baking sheet. Bake for 30-40 minutes.
- Heat olive oil in a pan, add garlic and shallot, and sauté until fragrant. Pour in tomato sauce, basil, oregano, and pepper. Simmer for 10-15 minutes.
- Scrape cooked spaghetti squash with a fork to create "noodles". Serve topped with tomato sauce. Serve As a pasta alternative with a side of steamed vegetables.

Cauliflower Fried Rice with Shrimp
Ingredients: 4 servings

1 lb. shrimp, peeled and deveined

1 head cauliflower, grated into rice-like pieces

1 cup mixed vegetables (such as peas, carrots, bell peppers)

2 cloves garlic, minced

2 eggs, beaten

3 tablespoons soy sauce

1 tablespoon sesame oil

2 green onions, chopped

Salt and pepper to taste

Procedure

- Heat sesame oil in a large skillet over medium heat. Add minced garlic and sauté until fragrant.
- Add shrimp and cook until pink and opaque. Remove from skillet and set aside.
- In the same skillet, add beaten eggs and scramble until cooked through. Remove from skillet and set aside. Add grated cauliflower and mixed vegetables to the skillet. Stir-fry until the cauliflower is tender.
- Return the cooked shrimp and scrambled eggs to the skillet. Stir in soy sauce and green onions. Cook for another minute. Season with salt and pepper before serving.

Veggie and Bean Burrito Bowl
Ingredients: 2 servings

2 cups cooked brown rice

1 can black beans, drained and rinsed

1 cup corn kernels

1 bell pepper, diced

½ red onion, diced

1 avocado, sliced

¼ cup chopped fresh cilantro

1 lime, cut into wedges

Optional toppings: salsa, Greek yogurt, shredded cheese

Procedure

- Divide cooked brown rice among serving bowls. Top with black beans, corn kernels, diced bell pepper, diced red onion, and chopped cilantro.
- Squeeze lime juice over the bowl and add the sliced avocado. Serve with optional toppings as desired.

Beef Stir-Fry with Broccoli and Mushrooms

Ingredients: 4 servings

1 lb. beef sirloin, thinly sliced

2 cups broccoli florets

1 cup sliced mushrooms

½ red bell pepper sliced

2 tablespoons low-sodium soy sauce

1 tomatoes diced

1 tablespoon cornstarch

2 cloves garlic, minced

½ cup low-sodium chicken broth

2 tablespoons vegetable oil (peanut)

Procedure

- Heat oil in a wok or skillet and sauté garlic until fragrant, add the vegetables and stir until tender, remove the vegetables and set aside.
- In the same skillet, stir fry the beef until cooked, and in a bowl mix soy sauce, cornstarch, and stock.
- Add the sauce, and tomatoes to the skillet and stir, add vegetables, and heat until the sauce is thick.
- Serve on rice.

Balsamic Glazed Pork Chops
Ingredients:

4 pork chops

¼ cup balsamic vinegar

2 tablespoons honey

2 cloves garlic, minced

1 teaspoon dried rosemary

¼ teaspoon dried thyme

Pepper to taste

Olive oil for cooking

1 small onion

4 ounces mushroom

1 teaspoon unsalted butter

Procedure

- In a small bowl, whisk together balsamic vinegar, honey, minced garlic, dried rosemary, and thyme pepper to make the glaze. Marinade the pork for some minutes.
- Heat olive oil in a skillet over medium-high heat. Add pork chops to the skillet and cook for 4-5 minutes on each side, or until browned and cooked through.
- Reduce heat to medium-low and pour the balsamic glaze over the pork chops in the skillet.
- Cook for an additional 2-3 minutes, allowing the glaze to thicken and coat the pork chops.
- Serve the pork chops hot, spooning any extra glaze from the skillet over the top.
- In the same skillet, add the butter, and sauté onion and mushroom until tender and mushroom browned.
- Serve alongside balsamic pork.

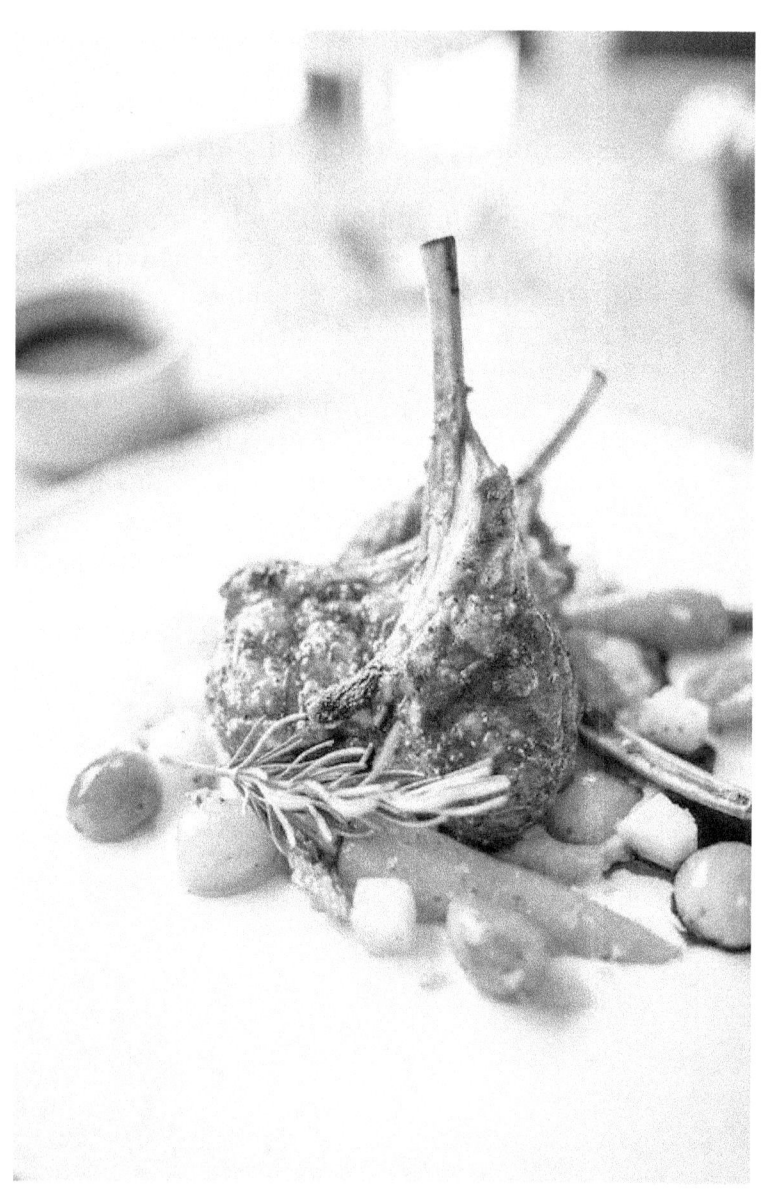

Coconut Rice Pudding

Ingredients: 4 servings

1 cup white rice (short or medium-grain)

4 cups coconut milk

¼ cup granulated sugar (or sugar substitute)

1 teaspoon vanilla extract

¼ cup shredded unsweetened coconut (optional)

Ground cinnamon for garnish (optional)

Procedure

- Till the water runs clear, rinse the rice under cold water. Place the rice and coconut milk in a saucepan. Over medium heat, bring it to a boil, and then turn down the heat.
- Cover and simmer for 20 to 25 minutes, stirring from time to time, or until the rice is soft and the mixture has thickened.
- Add the sugar, crushed coconut (if using), and vanilla essence. Cook the pudding for a further five to ten minutes, or until the consistency you like is reached. Turn off the heat and let it cool. Serve warm or cold, topped, if preferred, with ground cinnamon.

Lemon Blueberry Cheesecake Bites

Ingredients: 6-8 cheesecake bite

1 cup low-fat cream cheese

¼ cup Greek yogurt

Zest of 1 lemon

2 tablespoons fresh lemon juice

2-3 tablespoons honey or sugar substitute

½ teaspoon vanilla extract

Fresh blueberries for topping

Procedure

- In a mixing bowl, combine the low-fat cream cheese, Greek yogurt, lemon zest, lemon juice, honey (or sugar substitute), and vanilla extract. Mix until smooth and well combined. Spoon the cheesecake mixture into small serving cups or molds. Refrigerate for at least 2-3 hours to allow the cheesecake bites to set.

Note: you can enjoy this recipe with graham cracker crumbs by firstly mixing it with butter, spreading it in a baking dish, and baking for about five minutes, then scoop the mixture on the crust and refrigerate.

Carrot Cake Oatmeal Cookies:

Ingredients: 12-15 cookies

1 cup oats

½ cup grated carrots

1 cup all-purpose flour

½ cup unsalted butter

½ teaspoon baking soda

½ teaspoon baking powder

½ cup each granulated and brown sugar

¼ cup raisin

1 teaspoon lemon extract

1 large egg

½ teaspoon cinnamon

Procedure

- In a bowl, mix flour, baking powder, baking soda, and cinnamon.
- In a mixer, combine butter, and sugar until fluffy, add egg and lemon juice to combine thoroughly.
- Add flour mixture to the egg mixture and combine until blended, stir in the oat, carrot, and raisin. Combine thoroughly and leave for about 20 minutes.
- Preheat the oven to 350°F (175°C) and line a baking sheet with parchment paper.

- Form the mixture into cookies and place them on the prepared baking sheet. Bake for 12-15 minutes until golden brown. Allow cookies to cool before serving.

Mango Sorbet

Ingredients: **3-4 servings**

4 ripe mangoes, peeled and diced

¼ cup honey or sugar substitute

2 tablespoons fresh lime or lemon juice

½ cup water

Procedure

- Pour the diced mangoes into a food processor or blender, Add honey (or sugar substitute) and lime or lemon juice.
- Blend until smooth. If the mixture is too thick, add water gradually while blending until desired consistency is reached.
- Transfer the mixture to a shallow dish and freeze for 3-4 hours, stirring every 30 minutes to break up ice crystals until it's firm but scoopable. Once properly frozen, scoop into serving bowls or cones.

Almond Flour Chocolate Cake
Ingredients: 8-10 servings

2 cups almond flour

½ cup unsweetened cocoa powder

1 teaspoon baking soda

¼ teaspoon salt

½ cup unsweetened applesauce

¼ cup vegetable oil

¾ cup granulated sugar (or sugar substitute)

4 large eggs

1 teaspoon vanilla extract

Procedure

- Preheat oven to 350°F (175°C). Grease a cake pan. In a bowl, whisk together almond flour, cocoa powder, baking soda, and salt.
- In another bowl, mix applesauce, vegetable oil, sugar, eggs, and vanilla extract until well combined. Gradually add the dry and wet ingredients, stirring until thoroughly combined.
- Transfer the mixture to the ready-made cake pan. Bake for 30 to 35 minutes or when a toothpick put into the center comes out clean, after letting the cake set in the pan for 10 minutes, turn it out onto a wire rack to finish cooling.

Date and Walnut Bars

Ingredients: **8-10 bars**

1 cup pitted dates, chopped

¼ cup water

1 teaspoon vanilla extract

1 cup oat flour (finely ground oats)

½ teaspoon baking soda

¼ teaspoon salt

½ cup chopped walnuts

Procedure

- Set oven temperature to 175°C/350°F. A baking pan can be lined with parchment paper or greased. Add the water and chopped dates to a saucepan. Cook, stirring periodically, over medium heat until dates soften and take on the consistency of paste.
- Take it off the stove, mix in the vanilla essence, and allow it to cool a little. Combine the oat flour, baking soda, salt, and chopped walnuts in another basin.
- Mix the dry ingredients with the date mixture until a dough forms. Using the prepared baking pan, press the dough evenly.
- Bake until the edges are golden brown, 15 to 18 minutes. Let it cool down in the pan entirely before slicing into bars.

Gingerbread Cookies

Ingredients: **24 cookies**

2 cups all-purpose flour

1 teaspoon baking soda

1 teaspoon ground ginger

1 teaspoon ground cinnamon

¼ teaspoon ground cloves

½ cup unsalted butter, softened

½ cup brown sugar or granulated sugar

¼ cup molasses or honey

2 egg whites

Low-phosphorus icing (optional)

Procedure

- Combine the flour, baking soda, cloves, ginger, cinnamon, and salt in a bowl. Creamy butter and brown sugar should be combined in a separate basin.
- Beat the egg and molasses into the butter mixture thoroughly. Mixing until mixed, gradually add the dry ingredients to the wet ones.
- Split the dough in half, press the dough into discs, cover with plastic wrap, and chill for a minimum of two hours. Set oven temperature to 175°C/350°F. Use parchment paper to line baking sheets.

- Roll out the dough to a thickness of approximately 1/4 inch on a surface dusted with flour. Cut into the appropriate shapes using cookie cutters.
- Lay out cookies on baking sheets that have been prepped, and bake for 8 to 10 minutes, or until edges are hard. If you would like to decorate the cookies with low-phosphorus icing, wait until they are cool.

Honey Yogurt Parfait
Ingredients: 2 servings

2 cups low-fat Greek yogurt

¼ cup honey

1 cup mixed fresh berries (such as strawberries, blueberries, raspberries)

¼ cup low phosphorus granola

Procedure

- In a bowl, mix Greek yogurt and honey until well combined. In serving glasses or bowls, layer the honey yogurt mixture, fresh berries, and granola. Repeat the layers as desired, ending with a sprinkle of granola on top.

Avocado Chocolate Mousse
Ingredients: 4 servings

2 ripe avocados, peeled and pitted

¼ cup unsweetened cocoa powder

¼ cup honey or sugar substitute

1 teaspoon vanilla extract

Pinch of salt

Fresh berries for garnish (optional)

Procedure

- In a food processor or blender, combine the avocados, cocoa powder, honey (or sugar substitute), vanilla extract, and salt. Blend until smooth and creamy, scraping down the sides as needed to ensure everything is mixed well.
- Divide the chocolate mousse into serving cups or bowls. Refrigerate for at least 30 minutes to chill and serve. Before serving, garnish with fresh berries if desired.

Orange Almond Cake
Ingredients: 8-10 servings

1 ½ cups almond flour

½ cup granulated sugar (or sugar substitute)

Zest of 1 orange

½ teaspoon baking powder

¼ teaspoon salt

3 large eggs

¼ cup vegetable oil

2 tablespoons fresh orange juice

1 teaspoon vanilla extract

Procedure

- Preheat oven to 350°F (175°C). Grease a cake pan. In a bowl, whisk together almond flour, sugar, orange zest, baking powder, and salt.
- In another bowl, beat eggs, vegetable oil, orange juice, and vanilla extract until well combined. Add the dry ingredients to the wet components little by little and stir until just blended.
- Fill the prepared cake pan with the batter. Bake for about 30-35 minutes or until a toothpick inserted in the middle comes out clear.

Lemon Yogurt cake
Ingredients: 8–10 slices

1½ cups of flour for all purposes

½ cup almond flour

1 tsp. baking powder

½ tsp. baking soda

A pinch of salt

1 cup of Greek yogurt, plain

¾ cup of sugar, granulated

3 big eggs

Lemon zest of 1 lemon

¼ cup of newly squeezed lemon juice

½ teaspoon vanilla extract

¼ cup vegetable oil

Procedure

- Set oven temperature to 175°C/350°F. Apply grease to a loaf pan.
- Mix the flour, baking soda, baking powder, and salt in a bowl.
- Combine yogurt, sugar, eggs, lemon zest, lemon juice, vanilla extract, and vegetable oil in a separate bowl and whisk until thoroughly blended.
- Gradually add the dry ingredients to the wet ones, mixing just until combined. After the loaf pan is ready, pour the batter into it.
- A toothpick inserted into the center should come out clean after 45 to 50 minutes of baking.
- After letting the cake set in the pan for ten minutes, turn it out onto a wire rack to finish cooling.
- Garnish slices with fresh berries or a dollop of low-phosphorus whipped topping.

Angel Food Cake with Fresh Berries

Ingredients: **10-12 servings**

1 ¼ cups egg whites (about 9 large eggs)

1 cup granulated sugar

1 cup cake flour

1 teaspoon cream of tartar

1 teaspoon vanilla extract

Fresh berries (strawberries, blueberries, raspberries) for topping

Procedure

- Preheat oven to 350°F (175°C). In a large mixing bowl, beat egg whites until frothy.
- Add cream of tartar and continue beating until soft peaks form. Gradually add powdered sugar while continuing to beat until stiff peaks form. Gently fold in cake flour and vanilla extract until well combined.
- Pour the batter into an ungreased angel food cake pan. Bake for 35-40 minutes or until the top is lightly golden and the cake springs back when touched. Invert the pan onto a cooling rack and let it cool completely before removing the cake. Top slices of angel food cake with fresh berries before serving.

Pumpkin Spice Muffins
Ingredients: 10-12 muffins

1 cup all-purpose flour

¾ cup whole-wheat flour

1 teaspoon baking soda

½ teaspoon baking powder

½ teaspoon salt

1 teaspoon ground cinnamon

½ teaspoon ground nutmeg

½ teaspoon ground ginger

¼ teaspoon ground cloves

1 cup canned pumpkin puree

½ cup unsweetened applesauce

¼ cup vegetable oil

1 cup granulated sugar (or sugar substitute)

2 large eggs

1 teaspoon vanilla extract

Procedure

- Turn the oven on to 375°F, or 190°C. Use paper liners to line a muffin tray.
- Mix the flour, baking powder, baking soda, salt, cloves, nutmeg, and cinnamon in a basin.

- Pumpkin puree, applesauce, vegetable oil, sugar, eggs, and vanilla extract should all be thoroughly mixed in a separate basin.
- Mix the dry ingredients to the wet ones until incorporated thoroughly, Pour the mixture into the muffin tins.
- Bake for about 20-25 minutes or until toothpick or tester inserted inside out clean.

Banana Walnut Bread

Ingredients: **1 loaf (8-10 slices)**

3 ripe bananas, mashed

1/3 cup unsweetened applesauce

¼ cup vegetable oil

½ cup granulated sugar (or sugar substitute)

1 teaspoon vanilla extract

1 cups all-purpose flour

½ cup oat flour

1 teaspoon baking soda

¼ teaspoon salt

½ cup chopped walnuts

Procedure

- Preheat oven to 350°F (175°C). Grease a loaf pan. In a large bowl, mix mashed bananas, applesauce, vegetable oil, sugar, and vanilla extract.

- Mix the flour, baking soda, and salt in a separate bowl. Stirring until just blended, gradually add the dry ingredients to the wet components. Add the chopped walnuts and fold. Pour the batter into the set loaf pan.
- Bake for 50 -60 minutes or until the tester comes out clean when inserted in the middle.
- Allow the banana walnut bread to cool in the pan for 10 minutes before transferring it to a wire rack to cool completely.

Vanilla Panna Cotta with Raspberry Sauce

Ingredients: **4 servings**

2 cups low-fat milk

¼ cup granulated sugar (or sugar substitute)

1 teaspoon vanilla extract

2 teaspoons unflavored gelatin

2 tablespoons cold water

1 cup fresh or frozen raspberries

2 tablespoons water

1-2 tablespoons honey or sugar (optional)

Plain yogurt or whipped cream (optional)

Procedure

- In a saucepan, heat the milk and sugar over medium heat until it's warm but not boiling. Add in the vanilla extract and remove from heat.
- In a small bowl, sprinkle gelatin over cold water and let it sit for a few minutes to soften. Add the softened gelatin to the warm milk mixture and whisk until completely dissolved.
- Pour the mixture into individual serving cups or ramekins. Refrigerate for at least 2-4 hours or until set.
- For the raspberry sauce, in a small saucepan, combine raspberries, water, and honey or sugar (if using). Simmer over medium heat until the raspberries soften and the sauce starts to get somewhat thicker. Take off from heat and filter using a fine-mesh strainer to eliminate the seeds. After the panna cotta sets, drizzle the raspberry sauce over it.

Chia Seed Pudding

Ingredients   1 servings

¼ cup chia seeds

1 cup plant-based milk (coconut milk /almond milk)

1 tsp. vanilla extract

½ Tbsp. Maple syrup or honey

¼ tsp. cinnamon

1 tablespoon cocoa powder (optional)

Sliced fruit for topping (berries or banana)

Procedure

- Mix chia seeds with coconut milk, vanilla extract, cocoa if using, and a touch of maple syrup if using
- Stir well and refrigerate for at least two hours until it thickens or refrigerate overnight
- Once the pudding is set, layer it in serving cups or bowls, alternating with layers of low-phosphorus whipped topping and fresh or canned cherries. Garnish with additional cherries on top before serving.

Pineapple Upside-Down Cake

Ingredients: 8-10 servings

1 can pineapple slices in juice, drained or 1 whole pineapple peeled, cored, and cut in ring form.

¼ cup unsalted butter, melted (optional)

½ cup brown sugar (or sugar substitute)

Maraschino cherries, drained

1 ½ cups all-purpose flour

1 teaspoon baking powder

¼ teaspoon salt

½ cup unsweetened applesauce or milk

½ cup granulated sugar (or sugar substitute)

2 large eggs

1 teaspoon vanilla extract

Procedure

- Set oven temperature to 175°C/350°F. Oil a circular cake pan. Place the pineapple slices in the cake pan's bottom. Put a cherry in the middle of every slice of pineapple.
- Dust the pineapple slices and cherries with brown sugar. Pour melted butter over the top.
- Mix the flour, baking powder, and salt in a bowl. Combine applesauce, eggs, granulated sugar, and vanilla extract in a separate basin and whisk thoroughly.
- Mixing until mixed thoroughly, gradually add the dry ingredients to the wet ones. Over the pineapple slices in the pan, pour the batter.
- Bake for about 30-35 minutes or until the cake is set, let it cool for some minutes before turning it in the pan.

Lemon Ricotta Cookies
Ingredients: 24 cookies

2 cups all-purpose flour

½ teaspoon baking powder

½ teaspoon baking soda

¼ teaspoon salt

½ cup unsalted butter, softened

1 cup granulated sugar (or sugar substitute)

1 cup ricotta cheese

1 large egg

2 tablespoons fresh lemon juice

Zest of 1 lemon

Powdered sugar for dusting (optional)

Procedure

- Set oven temperature to 175°C/350°F. Use parchment paper to line baking sheets. Mix the flour, baking soda, baking powder, and salt in a bowl.
- Beat sugar and butter together in a separate dish until frothy and light. Stir in the egg, lemon zest, juice, and ricotta cheese. Blend until thoroughly blended. Mixing until mixed thoroughly, add the dry ingredients to the wet ones.
- Drop dough onto the prepared baking sheets by spoonful. Bake for 12 to 15 minutes, or until cookies are slightly brown around the edges and firm.
- After a few minutes, let the cookies cool on the baking sheets before moving them to a wire rack to finish cooling. If desired, dust with powdered sugar.

Chocolate Banana Bread

Ingredients: 1 loaf (8-10 slices)

3 ripe bananas, mashed

1/ cup unsweetened applesauce

¼ cup vegetable oil

2/3 cup granulated sugar

1 teaspoon vanilla extract

1 ¾ cups all-purpose flour

¼ cup unsweetened cocoa powder

1 teaspoon baking soda

½ teaspoon salt

½ cup semi-sweet chocolate chips

Procedure

- Preheat oven to 350°F (175°C). Grease a loaf pan. In a large mixing bowl, combine mashed bananas, applesauce, vegetable oil, sugar, and vanilla extract.
- In another bowl, whisk together flour, cocoa powder, baking soda, and salt. Add the dry ingredients to the wet components little by little and stir until just blended. Add the chocolate chips and fold.
- Fill the prepared loaf pan with the batter. Bake for about 50-60 minutes or until a toothpick inserted in the center comes out clean. After 10 minutes of cooling in the pan, move the bread to a wire rack to finish cooling.

Carrot Cake Muffins

Ingredients: 12 muffins

1 ½ cups grated carrots

½ cup whole wheat flour

½ cup all-purpose flour

½ cup rolled oats

1 teaspoon baking powder

½ teaspoon baking soda

1 teaspoon ground cinnamon

¼ teaspoon ground nutmeg

¼ teaspoon salt

½ cup unsweetened applesauce

¼ cup honey, maple syrup

¼ cup vegetable oil

2 large eggs

1 teaspoon vanilla extract

½ cup chopped walnuts (optional)

Procedure

- Set oven temperature to 175°C/350°F. Use paper liners to line a muffin tray.
- Flour, oats, baking soda, baking powder, nutmeg, cinnamon, and salt should all be combined in a basin.

- Combine applesauce, eggs, vegetable oil, honey or maple syrup, and vanilla extract in a separate bowl.
- Mix the dry and wet components until they are well blended. Stir in grated carrot, if using, fold in chopped walnuts, and distribute the batter among the muffin tins.
- When a toothpick put into the center comes out clean, bake for 18 to 20 minutes.

Blueberry and Spinach Smoothie:
Ingredients:

1 cup fresh or frozen blueberries

1 cup fresh spinach leaves

½ cup low-potassium yogurt

½ cup almond milk (unsweetened)

Procedure

- Wash the blueberries and spinach thoroughly. Add blueberries, spinach, low-potassium yogurt, and almond milk to a blender.
- On high speed until smooth and creamy, blend. Add more almond milk or water if smoothie is thick to reach your desired consistency

Cucumber and Mint Infused Water:
Ingredients:

Slices of cucumber

Fresh mint leaves

Water

Procedure

- Thinly slice a cucumber. Combine cucumber and mint in a pitcher of water and let it infuse in the fridge for a few hours. Serve over ice if desired.

Peachy Green Smoothie
Ingredients:

1 ripe peach, peeled and chopped

½ cup of spinach leaves

½ banana

¼ cup coconut water (avoid if watching potassium)

1 tablespoon of honey (optional)

½ cup of ice cubes

Procedure

- Blend all ingredients until smooth. Adjust sweetness with honey if desired. Serve chilled.

Banana Oat Smoothie
Ingredients:

1 ripe banana

¼ cup of rolled oats (cooked and cooled)

½ cup of unsweetened almond milk

1 tablespoon of almond butter

½ teaspoon of cinnamon

½ cup of ice cubes

Procedure

- Blend all ingredients until smooth. Add more almond milk to suit your desired consistency. Serve immediately.

Tropical Delight Smoothie

Ingredients:

½ cup of pineapple chunks (fresh or canned in juice)

½ banana

¼ cup of mango chunks (fresh or frozen)

½ cup of unsweetened coconut milk

½ cup of ice cubes

Procedure

- Blend all ingredients until smooth and creamy. Add more coconut milk if necessary. Serve chilled.

Cucumber Mint Cooler

Ingredients:

½ cucumber, peeled and chopped

¼ cup of fresh mint leaves

Juice of 1 lime

½ cup of unsweetened coconut water (avoid if watching potassium)

1 tablespoon of honey (optional)

½ cup of ice cubes

Procedure

- Blend cucumber, mint leaves, lime juice, coconut water, and honey until smooth. Add ice cubes and blend again until smooth.

Berry Blast Smoothie
Ingredients:

½ cup of mixed berries (strawberries, blueberries, raspberries)

½ cup of sliced apple

½ cup of low-potassium fruit juice (such as apple or cranberry juice)

¼ cup of plain Greek yogurt (low-fat)

½ cup of ice cubes

Procedure

- Blend all ingredients until smooth. Add water if necessary to achieve desired consistency. Serve immediately.

Herbal Tea

Ingredients:

Herbal tea bags (chamomile, peppermint, or rooibos)

Hot water

Lemon slices (optional)

Honey (optional)

Procedure

- Place the herbal tea bag in a cup. Pour hot water over the tea bag. Steep for the recommended time (usually 5-7 minutes). Remove the tea bag and discard. Sweeten with honey or stevia if desired

Avocado and Kale Smoothie

Ingredients:

1 ripe avocado, peeled and pitted

1 cup kale leaves, stems removed

Juice of ½ lemon

Water or low-potassium milk

Procedure

- Scoop out the flesh of the avocado and put it into a blender. Add the kale leaves and lemon juice. Pour in enough water or low-potassium milk to cover the ingredients. Blend until smooth and creamy. If the smoothie is too thick, add more liquid as needed.

Strawberry Banana Smoothie
Ingredients:

1 cup fresh or frozen strawberries

1 ripe banana

½ cup low-potassium milk (such as almond milk)

Ice cubes (optional)

Procedure

- Peel the banana and wash the strawberries. Add the strawberries, banana, low-potassium milk, and ice cubes (if using) to a blender. Blend until smooth and creamy.

Cranberry Spritzer
Ingredients:

½ cup unsweetened cranberry juice

1 tablespoon lemon juice

Raspberry sherbet

Sparkling water

Fresh lime slices

Procedure

- Pour cranberry juice, lemon juice, and raspberry sherbet into a glass and top with sparkling water. Add lime slices for extra flavor if desired and serve chilled in a tall glass.

Cherry Almond Smoothie
Ingredients:

1 cup frozen cherries

1 tablespoon almond butter

½ cup plain Greek yogurt

½ cup almond milk

1 ripe banana

Spinach (optional: and will change the color)

Procedure

- Blend all ingredients until smooth and serve chilled.

Pineapple Ginger Mocktail
Ingredients:

1 cup pineapple juice

1 teaspoon grated ginger

1 teaspoon maple syrup (optional)

Sparkling water (optional)

Procedure

- Mix pineapple juice and grated ginger. Add sparkling water if desired and serve chilled.

Carrot Orange Juice

Ingredients:

2 large carrots, peeled and chopped

2 oranges, peeled and segmented

1 apple or beet (optional)

Procedure

- Run the chopped carrots and orange segments through a juicer. Stir the juice to combine flavors. Serve immediately over ice if desired.

Beetroot and Berry Smoothie

Ingredients:

1 small beetroot, peeled and chopped

½ cup mixed berries (such as strawberries, blueberries, raspberries), and more for garnish.

½ cup mango

½ cup low-potassium milk (such as almond milk)

Pinch of cinnamon (optional)

Almonds for garnish

Procedure

- Place the chopped beetroot, mango, mixed berries, low-potassium milk, and a pinch of cinnamon in a blender. Blend until smooth and creamy.
- Add the garnish and ice cubes for a colder smoothie.

Celery and Pear Smoothie

Ingredients:

1 stalk of celery, chopped

1 ripe pear, cored and chopped

½ cup low-potassium yogurt

Ginger

1-2 tbsp. Lemon juice

Procedure

- Place the chopped celery, pear, ginger, lemon juice, low-potassium yogurt, and ice cubes in a blender. Blend until smooth and creamy. Adjust the thickness by adding more yogurt or ice cubes if needed. Pour into glasses and serve immediately.

Grapefruit juice

Ingredients

2 cups of fresh grapes (red or green)

½ medium pear

1 cup of water or desired quantity

1-2 tablespoons of honey or sweetener

1 teaspoon of lemon juice (optional, for added flavor)

Procedure

- Wash the grapes and pear, pour into the blender, and blend until smooth.
- Strain the mixture, add the sweetener, and stir until dissolved. Add the lemon if using and serve over ice or refrigerate.

Berry Hibiscus Iced Tea

Ingredients:

1 hibiscus tea bag

½ cup mixed berries (strawberries, raspberries, blueberries)

Ice cubes

Honey or stevia to taste (optional)

Procedure

- Steep the hibiscus tea bag in hot water according to package instructions. Once steeped, remove the tea bag and let the tea cool to room temperature.
- In a separate container, mash the mixed berries to release their juices. Fill a glass with ice cubes and add the mashed berries.
- Pour the cooled hibiscus tea over the ice and berries. Sweeten with honey or stevia if desired. Stir well and serve immediately.

Ginger Lemonade
Ingredients:

Juice of 1 lemon

1 teaspoon grated ginger

1 cup water

Honey or stevia to taste (optional)

Ice cubes

Procedure

- In a glass, combine the lemon juice and grated ginger. Add water and sweeten with honey or stevia if desired. Stir well until the ingredients are mixed. Add ice cubes to chill the lemonade. Stir again before serving.

Apple Cinnamon Smoothie:

Ingredients:

1 medium-sized apple, peeled, cored, and diced

½ cup low-potassium yogurt (such as Greek yogurt)

½ teaspoon ground cinnamon

¼ teaspoon vanilla extract

½ cup almond milk (unsweetened)

Ice cubes (optional)

Procedure

- Place the diced apple, low-potassium yogurt, ground cinnamon, vanilla extract, and almond milk in a blender. Add ice cubes if you prefer a colder smoothie.
- Blend until the mixture is smooth and creamy. Add more milk if thick to achieve the desired consistency.
- Taste and adjust the sweetness or cinnamon flavor as needed. Pour the smoothie into glasses and garnish with a sprinkle of cinnamon on top if desired.

Pineapple Protein Smoothie

Ingredients:

½ cup pineapple chunks (fresh or frozen)

½ cup low-potassium yogurt

¼ cup silken tofu or protein powder

½ cup unsweetened almond milk

1 tablespoon honey or maple syrup (optional)

Procedure

- In a blender, combine the pineapple chunks, low-potassium yogurt, silken tofu or protein powder, almond milk, and honey or maple syrup (if using). Add ice cubes if you prefer a colder smoothie.
- Blend until the mixture is smooth and creamy. Pour the smoothie into glasses and serve immediately.

Raspberry Chia Seed Jam

Ingredients: 1 jar

2 cups fresh raspberries

2 tablespoons honey or sugar substitute

2 tablespoons chia seeds

1 tablespoon fresh lemon juice

Procedure

- In a saucepan, cook raspberries and honey (or sugar substitute) over medium heat, stirring regularly, until the raspberries break down and turn syrupy.
- Mash the raspberries with a fork or potato masher.
- Stir in the chia seeds and lemon juice, then decrease the heat to low.
- Simmer for about 10-15 minutes, stirring often, until the sauce has thickened.
- Remove from heat and allow to cool. The jam will thicken as it cools.
- Place the jam in a jar or airtight container and chill. It will keep for around a week or can be frozen.

This recipe can be enjoyed as toppings for toast, desserts, or yogurts.

Baked Sweet Potato Fries

Ingredients:

2 sweet potatoes, cut into fries

1 tablespoon olive oil

½ teaspoon paprika

Procedure

- Preheat oven to 425°F (220°C). Toss sweet potato fries with olive oil and paprika, then spread on a baking sheet. Bake for 25-30 minutes until crispy.

Hummus with Vegetable Sticks

Ingredients:

1 can (15 ounces) chickpeas, drained

2 tbsp. tahini

2 tbsp. lemon juice

1 clove garlic, minced

2 tbsp. olive oil

Salt to taste

Carrot sticks for serving

Celery sticks for serving

Procedure

- Combine chickpeas, tahini, lemon juice, minced garlic, olive oil, and a pinch of salt in a food processor.
- Until smooth and creamy, add a little water to reach the desired consistency and blend.
- Transfer the hummus to a serving bowl and refrigerate until ready to serve. Serve with carrot sticks and celery sticks.

Roasted Chickpeas
Ingredients:

1 can of 15-ounce chickpeas, drained and rinsed

1 tablespoon olive oil

1 teaspoon paprika

½ teaspoon garlic powder

½ teaspoon cumin

½ teaspoon black pepper (optional)

Procedure

- Preheat oven to 400°F (200°C). Toss chickpeas with olive oil and spices, then spread on a baking sheet. Roast for 25-30 minutes or until crispy.

Cucumber Avocado Rolls

Ingredients:

1 cucumber

1 avocado

1 teaspoon lemon juice

1 tablespoon diced bell pepper or fresh herb

¼ teaspoon paprika

Procedure

- Peel the cucumber and slice it lengthwise into thick strips using a vegetable peeler. Mash the avocado and Spread mixed with lemon juice and pepper if desired on each strip, sprinkle with diced bell pepper, roll up, secure with a toothpick if desired, and sprinkle with paprika.

Cottage Cheese with Pineapple

Ingredients:

½ cup low-fat cottage cheese

½ cup diced fresh or canned in-juice pineapple

Chia seed for topping (optional)

Honey (optional)

Procedure

- Mix cottage cheese and diced pineapple, and sprinkle chia seed on top if needed.

Trail Mix
Ingredients:

1 cup unsalted almonds

1 cup unsalted cashews

1 cup unsalted pumpkin seeds

1 cup unsweetened dried cranberries

1 cup unsweetened dried apricots, chopped

½ cup unsweetened banana chips

½ teaspoon cinnamon (optional)

Procedure

- In a large mixing bowl, combine the almonds, cashews, pumpkin seeds, dried cranberries, chopped dried apricots, and banana chips.
- If desired, sprinkle cinnamon over the mix for added flavor. Toss the ingredients together until well combined.

Edamame Hummus
Ingredients:

1 cup shelled edamame, cooked

2 tablespoons tahini

2 tablespoons lemon juice

1 clove garlic, minced

2 tablespoons olive oil

Salt and pepper to taste

Whole grain crackers or veggie sticks.

Procedure

- Combine cooked edamame, tahini, lemon juice, minced garlic, olive oil, salt, and pepper in a food processor. Blend until smooth, adding a little water to achieve desired consistency.
- Serve with whole-grain crackers or vegetable sticks.

Rice Cake with Cottage Cheese and Berries
Ingredients:

1 rice cake

¼ cup low-fat cottage cheese

¼ cup mixed berries (such as strawberries, blueberries, and raspberries)

Procedure

- Spread cottage cheese evenly on the rice cake. Top with mixed berries.

Watermelon Feta Salad
Ingredients:

2 cups watermelon cubes

¼ cup crumbled feta cheese

½ medium onions sliced (optional)

1 tablespoon olive oil

1 tablespoon red wine vinegar

I tablespoon of lemon juice

Fresh mint leaves for garnish

Procedure

- In a bowl, combine watermelon cubes, onions, and crumbled feta cheese.
- Mix the liquid ingredients, add to the bowl, and gently toss to combine. Garnish with fresh mint leaves.

Tuna Cucumber Bites
Ingredients:

1 can (5 ounces) tuna, drained

1 cucumber, sliced (seedless)

2 tablespoons Greek yogurt

1 tablespoon chopped dill

½ onion diced (optional)

Ground pepper to taste

Procedure

- Mix tuna, Greek yogurt, onion, pepper, and dill. Place a spoonful of the tuna mixture on each cucumber slice.

Vegetable Crudités with Yogurt Dip

Ingredients:

Assorted vegetables (carrots, bell peppers, cucumber, etc.), sliced

1 cup plain Greek yogurt (low-fat)

1 teaspoon lemon juice

1 clove garlic, minced

Fresh or dry dill, and parsley

Salt and pepper to taste

Preparation

- Mix yogurt, lemon juice, minced garlic, fresh herbs, salt, and pepper in a bowl for the dip. Serve sliced vegetables with the yogurt dip.

Apple Cinnamon Oat Bars

Ingredients:

2 cups rolled oats

1 cup unsweetened applesauce

1 teaspoon vanilla extract

1 apple peeled and grated

¼ teaspoon baking soda

2 tablespoons unsalted butter

2 tablespoons honey

1 teaspoon cinnamon

Procedure

- Preheat oven to 350°F (175°C). Mix all ingredients in a bowl. Press mixture into a lined baking pan and bake for 20–25 minutes.

Roasted Cauliflower Popcorn
Ingredients:

1 head cauliflower, cut into florets

1 tablespoon olive oil

1 teaspoon garlic powder

1 teaspoon onion powder

1 teaspoon paprika

Sea salt to taste

Cracked pepper to taste

Preparation

- Preheat oven to 425°F (220°C). Toss cauliflower florets with olive oil, onion, paprika garlic powder, salt, and pepper.
- Spread on a baking sheet and roast for 20-25 minutes until golden brown

Baked Zucchini Chips

Ingredients:

2 zucchinis, thinly sliced

1 tablespoon olive oil

Paprika to taste

Cumin

Salt and pepper to taste

Hummus/ yogurt dip for serving

Procedure

- Preheat oven to 225°F (110°C). Toss zucchini slices with olive oil, paprika, cumin, salt, and pepper. Arrange in a single layer on a baking sheet and bake for 1-2 hours until crispy

Baked Kale Chips

Ingredients:

1 bunch of kale, stems removed and torn into pieces

1 tablespoon olive oil

Salt to taste

Procedure

- Preheat oven to 300°F (150°C).
- Toss and combine kale with olive oil and salt.
- Spread on a baking sheet and bake for 10-15 minutes until crisp.

Spinach Artichoke dip with Whole Wheat Pita Chips

Ingredients:

1 cup cooked spinach, chopped

½ cup artichoke hearts, chopped

½ cup Greek yogurt (optional)

¼ cup grated Parmesan cheese

1 -2 tablespoons lemon juice

2 green onion chopped

1 tablespoon olive oil

Pepper to taste

Whole wheat pita, cut into triangles and toasted

Procedure

- Mix chopped spinach, artichoke hearts, Greek yogurt, lemon juice, onion, pepper, oil, and Parmesan cheese. Allow to chill for about 5-8 hours or overnight
- Serve with toasted whole wheat pita chips.

Deviled Eggs
Ingredients:

2 large eggs

2 tablespoons low-fat mayonnaise

½ teaspoon Dijon mustard

1 ½ teaspoon pimento (canned) optional

½ teaspoon black pepper

Drops of white vinegar

Paprika for garnish (optional)

Chopped fresh chives for garnish (optional)

Procedure

- Bring the egg to a boil and cook, once cooked, cool and peel. Cut the eggs lengthwise and remove the yolk.
- Mash the egg yolk until smooth and mix with mayonnaise, mustard, black pepper, and vinegar. Mix until combined and creamy.
- Pipe or spoon the mixture inside the egg, sprinkle paprika and garnish with fresh chives if using.

Egg Salad Snacks
Ingredients:

4 large eggs

¼ cup low-fat mayonnaise/ sour cream

1 tablespoon Dijon mustard

½ medium onion chopped

1 tablespoon chopped fresh dill (optional)

1 tablespoon chopped fresh chives (optional)

Black pepper to taste

Whole wheat crackers, lettuce wraps, or low-sodium bread for serving

Procedure

- Hard boil the eggs, cool, and chop. Place in a bowl and add the onion, chopped dill, and chives if using.
- Mix in the cream, mustard, and black pepper in the egg bowl

Tofu Spring Rolls

Ingredients:

8 rice paper wrappers

1 block (14 oz.) firm tofu, drained & pressed

8 leaves romaine lettuce cut lengthwise

1 cup shredded cabbage

1 carrot, julienned

1 cucumber, julienned

¼ cup fresh mint leaves

¼ cup fresh cilantro leaves (optional)

¼ cup unsalted peanuts, chopped (optional, for garnish)

½ teaspoon black pepper

½ teaspoon cumin

Hoisin sauce or peanut sauce for dipping (choose low-sodium varieties if available)

Procedure

- Prepare tofu by cutting it into thin strips or cubes, whichever you prefer. Then season evenly with cumin and black pepper. Heat a non-stick skillet over medium heat. Add the tofu strips or cubes to the skillet and cook until lightly browned on all sides, about 5-7 minutes.
- Wash and prepare all the vegetables: shred the cabbage, julienne carrot, and cucumber. Pick the mint and cilantro leaves from their stems.
- Soften Rice Paper Wrappers by dipping them in boiled and warm water until they become soft and pliable.
- Assemble Spring Rolls by spreading the lettuce on the rice wrapper, then place a handful of cabbage on the bottom third of the rice wrapper. Add a few strips of cooked tofu, and layer on some juvenile carrots and cucumbers. Add a few fresh mints on top. Sprinkle chopped peanuts if desired.
- Fold the bottom edge of the rice paper wrapper over the filling, then fold in the sides, and roll tightly to enclose the filling like a burrito. Repeat the process with the remaining rice paper wrappers and filling ingredients until all

the filling is used up. Refrigerate and Serve the tofu spring rolls with hoisin sauce or peanut sauce for dipping.

Cranberry Dip with Fresh Fruit
Ingredients:

1 cup fresh or frozen cranberries

¼ cup honey or maple syrup

¼ teaspoon cinnamon

½ teaspoon nutmeg

1 teaspoon lemon juice

¼ cup water

8 ounces low-fat cream cheese, softened or sour cream

Assorted fresh fruits for dipping (apples, pears strawberries, and grapes)

Procedure

- To cook cranberry sauce, simmer cranberries and water until they burst, stir in honey, cinnamon and, nutmeg, simmer for 2-3 minutes.
- Make the dip by combining the sauce and the sour cream in a food processor and mix until combined. Refrigerate for at least 30 minutes.
- Cut fruits into bite size and toss apples with lemon juice to avoid browning.
- Arrange fruits on a platter and serve chilled dip alongside.

Tips to travel and eating out on the renal diet

Maintaining a renal diet while dining out or traveling can seem challenging, but with careful planning and awareness, it's entirely manageable. Whether you're exploring new culinary experiences or navigating unfamiliar territories, here are some tips to help you stick to your renal diet while enjoying your adventures:

Plan Ahead: Research restaurants or eateries at your destination that offer renal-friendly options. Many establishments now provide nutritional information online, allowing you to assess menu choices in advance.

Communicate Your Needs: Don't hesitate to inform your server about your dietary restrictions. Most restaurants are accommodating and can adjust dishes to suit your needs, such as substituting high-phosphorus ingredients with lower-phosphorus alternatives.

Focus on Fresh Ingredients: Opt for dishes made with fresh fruits, vegetables, lean proteins, and whole grains. These options are generally lower in sodium, potassium, and phosphorus compared to processed or pre-packaged foods.

Mind Your Portions: Pay attention to portion sizes, especially when dining out. Restaurant servings are often larger than what you might eat at home, so consider sharing a dish or asking for a half portion to avoid overeating.

Choose wisely: Look for menu items that align with renal diet guidelines, such as grilled or baked fish, skinless poultry, salads with vinaigrette dressing on the side, and steamed vegetables. Avoid dishes that are fried, heavily seasoned, or loaded with sauces, as they can be high in sodium and phosphorus.

Be Sodium Savvy: Request that your meal be prepared with less or no salt, or ask for sauces and dressings to be served on the side so you can control the amount you consume. Avoid adding extra salt to the table and steer clear of processed foods, which are often high in sodium.

Stay Hydrated: Traveling can be dehydrating, so be sure to drink plenty of fluids, preferably water. Limit your intake of sugary drinks and alcohol, as they can contribute to dehydration and may not be suitable for a renal diet.

Pack Snacks: Bring along renal-friendly snacks like unsalted nuts, fresh fruit, low-sodium crackers, or homemade trail mix to curb hunger between meals and avoid relying on less suitable options available on the go.

Consult a Dietitian: If you're unsure about what to eat or need personalized guidance, consider consulting a renal dietitian before your trip. They can provide tailored recommendations and help you create a meal plan that fits your dietary needs and travel itinerary.

Enjoy in Moderation: While it's important to adhere to your renal diet, it's also essential to enjoy your dining and travel experiences. Allow yourself the occasional indulgence but strive for balance and moderation to support your overall health and well-being.

By following these tips and staying mindful of your dietary requirements, you can savor delicious meals and explore new destinations while successfully managing your renal diet. Bon appétit and safe travels!

TIPS TO HELP YOU STICK TO YOUR RENAL DIET

Sticking to a renal diet can be challenging, but there are several strategies to help you stay on track:

Education and Understanding: Learn as much as you can about your condition and the dietary guidelines. Understanding why certain foods are restricted or recommended can make it easier to adhere to the diet.

Meal Planning: Plan your meals. This helps ensure you have the right ingredients on hand and reduces the temptation to stray from your diet when hunger strikes.

Seek Professional Guidance: Work closely with a registered dietitian or a healthcare professional specializing in renal nutrition. They can provide personalized advice and meal plans tailored to your specific needs.

Portion Control: Pay attention to portion sizes. Even foods that are considered healthy can be problematic if consumed in large quantities. Use measuring cups or a food scale if needed.

Food Journaling: Keep a food diary to track what you eat and how it affects your health. This can help identify patterns and make necessary adjustments to your diet.

Gradual Changes: If the diet requires significant changes from your current eating habits, consider making gradual adjustments. It can be less overwhelming and easier to sustain in the long term.

Support System: Share your dietary goals with friends, family, or a support group. Having a support system can provide encouragement and accountability.

Explore Variety: Find creative ways to prepare meals within the dietary restrictions. Experiment with new recipes, flavors, and cooking methods to prevent boredom with the limited choices.

Healthy Substitutions: Identify and incorporate healthy substitutions for restricted foods. For example, replacing high-sodium seasonings with herbs and spices or choosing healthier cooking methods like baking or grilling instead of frying.

Stay Hydrated: Proper hydration is crucial for kidney health. Monitor your fluid intake as advised by your healthcare professional.

Manage Stress: Stress can impact eating habits. Find stress-relieving activities like meditation, yoga, or hobbies to help manage stress levels and avoid stress-induced eating.

OPTIONS FOR CELEBRATION ON RENAL DIET

Celebrations are a time for joy and togetherness, often accompanied by delicious food. For individuals following a renal diet, it's important to maintain balance while still enjoying the festivities. Here are some renal-friendly options suitable for celebrations:

Grilled Chicken Skewers: Marinate chicken chunks in a low-sodium herb marinade and grill them for a flavorful protein option.

Vegetable Platter with Hummus: Offer a colorful array of sliced vegetables like carrots, cucumbers, bell peppers, and cherry tomatoes served with kidney-friendly hummus.

Quinoa Salad: Prepare a quinoa salad with chopped cucumbers, tomatoes, bell peppers, and parsley, dressed with a light vinaigrette. Quinoa is a great protein and fiber source.

Fruit Salad: Create a refreshing fruit salad using kidney-friendly fruits like apples, berries, grapes, and pineapple. Avoid high-potassium fruits like oranges and bananas.

Shrimp Cocktail: Serve chilled shrimp with a side of low-sodium cocktail sauce for a tasty appetizer.

Vegetable Soup: Prepare a homemade vegetable soup using low-sodium broth, assorted vegetables, and herbs for flavor.

Grilled Fish Fillets: Season fish fillets with herbs and spices, then grill or bake them for a heart-healthy main dish rich in omega-3 fatty acids.

Rice Pilaf: Cook rice with low-sodium broth and add sautéed onions, garlic, and herbs for a flavorful side dish.

Greek Yogurt Dip: Make a creamy dip using Greek yogurt mixed with herbs and spices, served with raw vegetable sticks or whole-grain crackers.

Mocktail Bar: Offer a variety of kidney-friendly mocktails using sparkling water, fresh fruit juices, and garnishes like mint or citrus slices.

Tips on tasty food without salt

Herbs and Spices: Experiment with various herbs and spices to add depth and complexity to your dishes. Use fresh herbs like parsley, basil, cilantro, or mint, and spices such as cumin, paprika, turmeric, and garlic powder to season your food.

Citrus Zest and Juice: Citrus fruits like lemons, and limes, can bring brightness and tanginess to your meals. Use their zest and juice to enhance the flavor of salads, meats, and vegetables.

Vinegar: Balsamic, apple cider, and other flavored vinegar can add a pleasant acidity to dishes. Use them sparingly to avoid overpowering the flavors.

Onion and Garlic: These aromatic vegetables can significantly enhance the taste of your dishes.

Experiment with sautéing or roasting them to bring out their natural sweetness.

Homemade Stocks and Broths: Make your stocks using herbs, vegetables, and bones (if allowed in your diet) to create a flavorful base for soups, stews, and sauces.

Herb Blends and Marinades: Create custom herb blends or marinades using a combination of your favorite spices, herbs, and acidic ingredients like vinegar or citrus juice to marinate meats and vegetables.

Umami-rich Ingredients: Incorporate umami-rich foods like mushrooms, tomatoes, and miso paste to add depth and savory flavors to your dishes.

Fresh Ingredients: Use fresh, high-quality ingredients to bring out natural flavors. Ripe tomatoes, sweet bell peppers, and other fresh produce can add sweetness and depth to your meals.

Avoid Pre-Packaged and Processed Foods: Processed foods often contain high amounts of sodium. Opt for fresh, whole foods that you can season yourself.

MEASUREMENT CONVERSION CHART

1 teaspoon (tsp.) = 5 milliliters (ml)

1 tablespoon (tbsp.) = 3 teaspoons = 15 milliliters

1 fluid ounce = 2 tablespoons = 30 milliliters

1 cup = 8 fluid ounces = 16 tablespoons = 240 milliliters

1 pint = 2 cups = 16 fluid ounces = 480 milliliters

1 quart = 4 cups = 32 fluid ounces = 960 milliliters

1 gallon = 4 quarts = 16 cups = 128 fluid ounces = 3.8 liters

Weight Measurements:

1 ounce (oz.) = 28.35 grams (g)

1 pound (lb.) = 16 ounces = 453.59 grams

1 kilogram (kg) = 2.205 pounds = 1000 grams

Common Kitchen Equivalents:

1 stick of butter = 1/2 cup = 113.4 grams

1 standard US cup of flour = 120 grams

1 standard US cup of granulated sugar = 200 grams

1 standard US cup of water = 240 milliliters = 240 grams

1 clove of garlic = approximately 1 teaspoon minced

CONCLUSION

This cookbook is more than a collection of recipes—it's a guide to culinary creativity within the boundaries of a renal diet by harnessing the power of flavors, innovative ingredient swaps, and mindful cooking techniques, this book empowers individuals to savor every bite while nurturing their well-being.

Navigating a renal diet as an adult can present its challenges, but it's important to remember that you're not alone in this journey. By making mindful choices and staying committed to your health, you have the power to manage your condition effectively and live a fulfilling life.

Remember that every step you take towards following your renal diet is a step towards better health and well-being. Embrace the opportunity to explore new foods, flavors, and recipes that nourish your body while also bringing joy to your meals. Celebrate your progress, no matter how small, and recognize the strength and resilience within you.

Though there may be moments of frustration or uncertainty along the way, know that you have a support system of healthcare professionals, loved ones, and communities ready to assist you. Don't hesitate to reach out for guidance, encouragement, or simply a listening ear whenever you need it.

Above all, be kind to yourself and acknowledge the effort you're putting into taking care of your health. Each day presents an opportunity to make positive choices and move closer to your goals. Stay motivated, stay hopeful, and remember that with perseverance and determination, you can overcome any obstacle that comes your way.

You've got this. Keep shining bright on your journey to better health.

HAPPY COOKING!

7-day meal plan and free meal planning pages.

MEAL PLAN WEEK 1

MONDAY
Breakfast: quinoa porridge
Lunch: vegetable stir fry
Dinner: tilapia with mango salsa
Snacks/ dessert: mango sorbet

TUESDAY
Breakfast: vegetable omelets
Lunch: cauliflower rice stir fry
Dinner: chicken and broccoli Alfredo
Snacks/ dessert: honey yogurt parfait

WEDNESDAY
Breakfast: sweet potato breakfast hash
Lunch: chicken and vegetable lettuce wraps
Dinner: veggie lentil burger
Snacks/ dessert: angel food cake

THURSDAY
Breakfast: buckwheat pancakes
Lunch: turkey and vegetable skillet
Dinner: sweet potato and black bean quesadillas
Snacks/ dessert: orange almond cake

FRIDAY
Breakfast: chia seed pudding
Lunch: shrimp and vegetable skewers
Dinner: Greek yogurt chicken salad
Snacks/ dessert: lemon blueberry cheesecake

SATURDAY
Breakfast: egg white vegetable scramble
Lunch: vegetable and tofu stir fry
Dinner: turkey meatballs
Snacks/ dessert: carrot cake muffins

SUNDAY
Breakfast: spinach and feta frittata
Lunch: turkey and black bean tacos
Dinner: mushroom and spinach pasta
Snacks/ dessert: chocolate banana bread

MEAL PLAN WEEK 2
MONDAY
Breakfast:
Lunch:
Dinner:
Snacks/ dessert:

TUESDAY
Breakfast:
Lunch:
Dinner:
Snacks/ dessert:
WEDNESDAY
Breakfast:
Lunch:
Dinner:
Snacks/ dessert:

THURSDAY
Breakfast:
Lunch:
Dinner:

Snacks/ dessert:

FRIDAY
Breakfast:
Lunch:
Dinner:
Snacks/ dessert:

SATURDAY
Breakfast:
Lunch:
Dinner:
Snacks/ dessert:

SUNDAY
Breakfast:
Lunch:
Dinner:
Snacks/ dessert:

MEAL PLAN WEEK 3
MONDAY
Breakfast:
Lunch:
Dinner:
Snacks/ dessert:

TUESDAY
Breakfast:
Lunch:
Dinner:
Snacks/ dessert:

WEDNESDAY

Breakfast:
Lunch:
Dinner:
Snacks/ dessert:

THURSDAY
Breakfast:
Lunch:
Dinner:
Snacks/ dessert:

FRIDAY
Breakfast:
Lunch:
Dinner:
Snacks/ dessert:

SATURDAY
Breakfast:
Lunch:
Dinner:
Snacks/ dessert:

SUNDAY
Breakfast:
Lunch:
Dinner:
Snacks/ dessert:

MEAL PLAN WEEK 4

MONDAY
Breakfast:
Lunch:
Dinner:

Snacks/ dessert:

TUESDAY
Breakfast:
Lunch:
Dinner:
Snacks/ dessert:

WEDNESDAY
Breakfast:
Lunch:
Dinner:
Snacks/ dessert:

THURSDAY
Breakfast:
Lunch:
Dinner:
Snacks/ dessert:

FRIDAY
Breakfast:
Lunch:
Dinner:
Snacks/ dessert:

SATURDAY
Breakfast:
Lunch:
Dinner:
Snacks/ dessert:

SUNDAY
Breakfast:

Lunch:
Dinner:
Snacks/ dessert:

MEAL PLAN WEEK 5

MONDAY

Breakfast:
Lunch:
Dinner:
Snacks/ dessert:

TUESDAY

Breakfast:
Lunch:
Dinner:
Snacks/ dessert:

WEDNESDAY

Breakfast:
Lunch:
Dinner:
Snacks/ dessert:

THURSDAY

Breakfast:
Lunch:
Dinner:
Snacks/ dessert:

FRIDAY

Breakfast:
Lunch:
Dinner:
Snacks/ dessert:

SATURDAY

Breakfast:
Lunch:
Dinner:
Snacks/ dessert:

SUNDAY

Breakfast:
Lunch:
Dinner:
Snacks/ dessert:

MEAL PLAN WEEK 6

MONDAY

Breakfast:
Lunch:
Dinner:
Snacks/ dessert:

TUESDAY

Breakfast:
Lunch:
Dinner:
Snacks/ dessert:

WEDNESDAY

Breakfast:
Lunch:
Dinner:
Snacks/ dessert:

THURSDAY

Breakfast:
Lunch:
Dinner:
Snacks/ dessert:

FRIDAY

Breakfast:
Lunch:
Dinner:
Snacks/ dessert:

SATURDAY

Breakfast:
Lunch:
Dinner:
Snacks/ dessert:

SUNDAY

Breakfast:
Lunch:
Dinner:
Snacks/ dessert:

MEAL PLAN WEEK 7

MONDAY
Breakfast:
Lunch:
Dinner:
Snacks/ dessert:

TUESDAY
Breakfast:
Lunch:
Dinner:
Snacks/ dessert:

WEDNESDAY
Breakfast:
Lunch:
Dinner:
Snacks/ dessert:

THURSDAY
Breakfast:
Lunch:
Dinner:
Snacks/ dessert:

FRIDAY
Breakfast:
Lunch:
Dinner:
Snacks/ dessert:

SATURDAY
Breakfast:
Lunch:

Dinner:
Snacks/ dessert:

SUNDAY
Breakfast:
Lunch:
Dinner:
Snacks/ dessert:

www.ingramcontent.com/pod-product-compliance
Lightning Source LLC
Chambersburg PA
CBHW071043290526
45795CB00004B/1296